Know Your Body

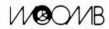

This book has been endorsed by
World Organization Ovulation Method-Billings,
U.S.A. and International

Know Your Body

A Family Guide to Sexuality and Fertility

Charles W. Norris, M.D.   Jeanne B. Waibel Owen, B.A.

OUR SUNDAY VISITOR, Inc.

HUNTINGTON

To the Divine Author of all,
with humility and gratitude,
and to our earthly spouses,
Carol and John

Editor
Paul Zomberg

Illustrator
James McIlrath

Designer
Paul Zomberg

ISBN 0-87973-658-5   LC Number 82-060666

PRINTED IN THE UNITED STATES OF AMERICA

Contents

Acknowledgments

To give sufficient credit to all who have helped us in bringing this book into existence would be as difficult as was the writing of it. There are many to whom we owe a special debt, for they not only guided us during all the stages of writing, but also gave us needed encouragement to continue.

In particular, we are indebted to the following persons and organizations:

To the board of directors of World Organization Ovulation Method-Billings, U.S.A.—Drs. John and Evelyn Billings, Mrs. Mercedes Wilson, Mrs. Margaret McGauley, Dr. John Brennan, Mrs. Marge Harrigan, and Mrs. Ann O'Donnell.

To the members of the Human Sexuality and Fertility Awareness Subcommittee of W.O.O.M.B., U.S.A.—Dr. Hanna Klaus, Dr. George Maloof, Dr. Ruth Taylor, Sister Anne Boessen, Mrs. Mary Therese Egizio, Sister Louise Marie Bryan, Mary Ursula Fagan, A.C.S.W., Mrs. Mary Thormann, and Mrs. Beattie Muraski—for their helpful comments, suggestions, and criticisms.

To the many families in Oregon who participated in extensive field-testing of an early draft of the book, and whose comments and suggestions led to many improvements in the text of the book.

To those who consented to read and criticize the text when it was in galleys, for their exceptionally useful comments and suggestions—Thomas J. O'Donnell, S.J., Mrs. Mary Rosera Joyce, Mr. John Harrington, Dr. Thomas W. Hilgers, Sister Marilyn Mangus, Dr. T. Glenn Haws, Mrs. Judie Brown, Mrs. Terrie Lee Guay, Dr. William Walsh, and Dr. James J. Pattee.

To Dr. and Mrs. Frank Ayd and their granddaughter Susan, who drew the frontispiece.

To our editor, Mr. Paul G. Zomberg, who saw the value of what we wanted to accomplish with this book, and who acted as midwife on our behalf to bring the book to publication.

And to our families, who suffered patiently with us during the many months when we struggled to bring a difficult undertaking to a happy conclusion.

C. W. N. / J. B. W. O.

A woman's reproductive system, as drawn by a nine-year-old girl.

Introduction

THIS IS A BOOK for young people entering adolescence and for their parents to share, to talk about, and to learn from. The subject of this book is human sexuality in the broad sense—whatever makes you a man or a woman—as well as in the limited sense of human reproductive organs. We will speak primarily to the young reader, attempting to answer the many questions that young people have about their own personal sexuality and fertility. If by chance we do not answer every question that every reader brings to this book, perhaps we will have managed to answer at least some of the more important questions—including some questions that we have only recently learned to ask.

We wrote this book after becoming aware of the several ways in which young people are being misguided about their sexuality. We saw that young people are often left to themselves in coping with it, without accurate information or good counsel.

In our society, "sexual freedom" is promoted as a desirable thing. But such freedom has resulted in increasing the number of unwed pregnant teenage girls (more than a million in 1980) and the spread of sexually transmitted diseases (venereal diseases). In some schools, students in health classes are told

1

by their teachers that parents, having been raised in a different era with different moral standards, are not the best source of up-to-date information about sexuality. We think that parents are precisely the persons to whom growing children can and should go for information about all the important things in human life, including sexual things. We hope this book will enable parents and their older children to make sexuality one of the "important things" they can discuss honestly, privately, and without embarrassment.

We do not intend that the information in this book be forced on any child. In every child's life, there comes an ideal time—and it *may* be sooner than many parents think—to learn everything in this book. Actually, we have included in our chapters more information than might have been required for some readers, and less than others would like to have; but we have tried to answer all the questions that young people commonly ask about their sexuality, as well as provide them with the information we think every person needs in order to be sexually responsible. We ask the readers of this book to keep in mind that there are many aspects of human sexuality that we do not touch on—either through oversight or because we thought those aspects were outside the scope of what we hoped to accomplish. To help those who need further information or guidance about human sexuality, we have included a list of books we can recommend.

We suspect that many readers will find it fairly difficult to understand some parts of this book on first reading. Some of the topics we discuss are quite technical and require the use of several technical terms. At the end of the book, we include a glossary of terms that are likely to be unfamiliar. Terms that appear in **bold face type** are among those listed in the Glossary; these terms especially need to be understood.

We also include a list of questions that we think a young person needs to be able to answer if he or she is to be properly informed about his or her sexuality and fertility. Parents reading this book for the first time might well look over those questions before reading the chapters themselves; for parents too need to be well informed if they are to be the source of information and guidance for their children.

It is a natural role of parents to guide their children safely through the transition called adolescence. They should look upon this book as *one* of the ways in which they can help their children become men and women who accept their sexuality, appreciate their powers of fertility, and are ready to make a free and unconditional commitment of themselves in marriage if that is their vocation.

In families where parents are good listeners to their children, education in sexuality happens gradually and naturally. We hope this book will supplement that kind of listening where it exists, and encourage it where it has not been common. It is one of the great joys of parenthood, we think, to see one's children grow toward adulthood and be able to share in adult conversations.

We should add here that, over the years, we have noticed that when we have spoken to families about *fertility* rather than about *sex,* there has been a noticeable absence of embarrassment; instead, young people especially find it fascinating to learn about their fertility, as a key to their sexuality. When they understand their fertility, they gain a deeper appreciation of their sexuality. Parents who respect and appreciate their own fertility are the ideal persons to pass these attitudes on to their children.

The values of human fertility are also the values of human sexuality. A man who despises (or treats lightly) his fertility also despises (or treats as a plaything) something of what makes him a man; and so also for a woman and her femininity. One finds recent medical textbooks discussing both fertility and infertility as *undesirable conditions,* even as diseases, and one wonders how young people can make sense of their sexuality in a society that treats it as a medical problem or as a plaything.

It is *as a male* or *as a female* that each of us is a human being. We wish for our readers, especially those who are beginning to discover themselves as men or women, that they accept their sexuality, welcome their sexual maturing, and love everything that makes them sexual beings. Adolescence will bring to each young person a spurt in physical growth and change, as well as a certain amount of emotional upset, so that one needs time to cope with a "new self" that sometimes appears almost from day to day. It is fairly common for teenagers to dislike themselves and to wish they were other people.

We hope this book will help young people to prepare themselves for such moments and survive them, knowing that the day is coming when they will look in a mirror and begin to admire themselves for who they are. In the meantime, parents can be understanding and steadfastly affirm the goodness of their children. Our goal, in the following pages, is to affirm the goodness of human sexuality, and to help young people affirm it also.

In each chapter of this book, we have tried to summarize many things briefly but clearly. Most readers of the book can think of it as a "good start" toward obtaining the information they need to know about their sexuality as men or women, and about their fertility. We have not spoken much about the subject of pregnancy and childbirth—a subject that would require another book. Nor have we spoken about marriage as such, or about the sexual relationship between husband and wife. Engaged couples should obtain appropriate counseling about these matters as they prepare for their wedding day. We have limited ourselves to providing young persons entering on puberty with the information they need in order to understand their own sexuality and fertility, whether they ever marry or not.

We like to think that if young people are able to see the connection between their sexuality and their fertility, they will value both as they should, and even pride themselves on their maturing sense of why God has made them male or female. Men should take pride in their manhood; women, in their womanhood. It is as a man or as a woman that each of us is expected to give an account of our lives in this world.

True, our sexuality is something that none of us ever fully understands. In medical terms, our reproductive systems are marvelous; in spiritual terms, they are mysterious. We hope this book helps young people to appreciate better both the marvelousness and the mystery.

Charles W. Norris
Jeanne B. Waibel Owen

CHAPTER ONE

Growing Older, Growing Up

GROWING OLDER is what happens automatically, with the passing of days, months, and years. Growing up is different, not automatic, not even always easy. You can look back and see how much you have "grown up." In one way, you can see that you are the same person you always were; but in another way, you are just as sure that you have changed, are different, from the child you used to be.

Little children have very strange ideas about grown-ups. They think grown-ups (such as their parents) have status and power, and have no one "bossing them around." As they reach the age of 8 or 9 or 10, those same children commonly wish they were teenagers. In their eyes, teenagers are fascinating people who lead interesting lives and wear neat clothes. They know what teenagers are on the outside. They don't know what it's like to be a teenager *on the inside.* You may know what *that* feels like—or at least you are beginning to know.

Perhaps you have read some books about teenage heroes and heroines that gave you a glimpse of what to expect during your own years as a teenager. One of the things you and every other teenager can expect is that your feelings will sometimes "get ahead of you," sometimes "take over." Most teenagers go through periods of thinking and feeling they are ugly or shunned or incompetent or manipulated or ridiculed or even sick; at other times, they may feel strongly loving, loyal, righteous, ambitious, and romantic. All such feelings are normal and typical. The little child cannot appreciate them; and the grown-ups in your life may sometimes get exasperated by your ups and downs—and you have to live with yourself!

Growing up means many things and can be measured in various ways. Each of us is born entirely dependent on others for our survival. In infancy, each of us looked to parents for love, training, reassurance, and a sense of order. We each noticed changes that affected us, ignored those that did not (such as the change in our mother's body during a subsequent pregnancy). We noticed when we could finally reach that doorknob or faucet all by ourselves, when we had to wear larger shoes, and when we were old enough to go to school. We learned how to get along with other children our own age, how to play and fight and share with them. Our good manners earned praise, and in time we became accustomed to dealing with a wider circle of people. We also grew in the sense or understanding we had of ourselves and our relationships to all the other people we knew.

When adolescence came upon us, we could look back and see that we were no longer helpless infants; but at the same time we found that we would have to double-check all our old understandings before we could get on to becoming fully independent persons, responsible to ourselves, for ourselves.

Because teenagers often find themselves thinking about themselves, they are likely to forget that the other members of their families have selves too! Every person in a family needs affection, needs to be helped, needs someone to listen to him or her, has worries and fears and emotions to deal with, and can be hurt just as easily as any teenager. Nothing about adolescence is entirely unique. All teenagers go through pretty much the same dramatic changes that adolescence brings. To be thirteen years old—suddenly a *teen*-ager—is not a tragedy; it would make more sense to think of it as a blessing, or even as an escape from childhood or childishness, a beginning of something better.

The physical changes associated with adolescence usually begin well before one's thirteenth birthday. It is perhaps unfortunate that we have gotten into the habit of setting teenagers apart as strange creatures who are neither children nor adults. Adolescence usually begins before we enter our teen years and continues after we leave them. Teenagers are persons caught in the middle of adolescence.

To make matters more confusing, neither boys nor girls all change in the same ways or at the same ages. (*See the chart on page 10.*) Even looking ahead to the changes of **puberty** (*PYOO-bir-tee*) and the period of adolescence does not always help: if you are a girl, you may wonder how large your breasts will grow; and if you are a boy, you may think you are not growing tall enough, fast enough. You are constantly comparing yourself to others your age; you are very conscious of the way you look, and you may or may not be sure you like what you see when you look at yourself in a mirror. One of the more difficult tasks you have is remembering that what you see in a mirror *is not necessarily what others see*; and it is also hard to keep in mind that what you see is a temporary, half-finished image of the new you.

Medical science does not clearly know what causes the increased secretions of **sex hormones** that begin the changes of puberty. After several years of slow and steady growth, there is a sudden growth spurt as puberty begins. So dramatic are its effects that young persons can go through a period of feeling that they no longer know who they are. For boys especially there can be a change in height so rapid and sudden that their clothes become too small in a matter of weeks. One needs to have some confidence that nature has things under control—that the changes are natural, and that they have a purpose.

Bodily Changes Typical of Adolescence

CHANGES IN GIRLS

• A fast gain in height may begin at about age 10; growth in height after a girl's first **menstruation** is typically 2 or 3 inches. The fastest growth rate may occur about age 12.

• The contour of the breasts takes form rapidly, along with growth of pubic hair and underarm hair.

• The first menstruation (menarche) occurs about a year after growth of the breasts.

• Menstrual cycles may occur without **ovulation** for a year or two after the first menstruation. Those cycles would *not* include a fertile phase.

• Menstrual cycles may be very irregular for a few years.

CHANGES IN BOYS

• A fast gain in height may begin at about age 12. The fastest growth-rate may occur anywhere between ages 10 and 16, but in most cases takes place near age 14.

• The first sign of pubertal change is sweating of feet and underarms.

• The testicles increase in size and become more sensitive to pressure.

• The scrotal sac containing the testicles becomes wrinkled, reddish.

• The penis becomes larger.

• Pubic hair, body hair, and facial hair appear.

• The voice changes to a lower pitch.

When a girl begins to menstruate (we discuss this subject in detail in a later chapter), she has evidence that her body is changing from that of a girl to that of a woman. She knows the onset of **menstruation** is an experience she shares with all other women, and she may welcome this sign of her maturing; but still it may bring a range of emotions to deal with. She needs to decide how she feels about this change in herself. If none of her girlfriends have yet started menstruating, she may well feel uncomfortable or even embarrassed about it at first. The same sort of discomfort can occur if she sees that her breasts have already become noticeably larger than those of other girls her age, *or* that other girls are ahead of her in breast development.

Boys who are experiencing the first changes of puberty have their own special changes to deal with. For example, as their bodies begin to mature, they find that they have spontaneous erections—that is, the tissues of the penis become filled with blood, and the penis becomes stiff and firm. An erection can be quite painful if clothing is tight. Boys are naturally self-conscious when an erection occurs spontaneously while others are present; they may fear that others will notice their plight. They may be proud of this evidence of their masculinity, but they may also fear being ridiculed about it. The appearance of facial hair, on the other hand, is similarly a sign of masculinity for adolescent boys, but causes little more than minor embarrassment and is perhaps the occasion for some goodnatured teasing from family and friends.

Of course, all of the changes that come with puberty have something to do with physical maturity—with your body's continuing the "building" that has gone on since the moment of your conception in your mother's body. Because you are, like every other person, either male or female, you are becoming very aware of your sexuality. But because there is not much that can be done to hurry or slow the rate of change, a certain amount of patience and a sense of humor are helpful in dealing with yourself and with others.

Puberty marks the time in your life when you become capable of being a father or a mother. This ability—or power—places upon you a very serious responsibility. Before we look more closely at that responsibility, we will explain, in the next chapter, what is involved in the sexuality of men and women. ☐

CHAPTER TWO

Human Sexuality

HAVING SEEN in a general way how the period of adolescence brings changes to every person, let's consider what human sexuality is, both in the broad sense of being male or female, and in the more limited sense of male and female reproductive organs.

Sexuality as Part of Human Nature

Each of us is a sexual being from the moment of our conception. At that moment, we are created biologically male or female. When each of us was born, our parents wanted to know whether we were "boy or girl." The answer to their question established our own sexual identity for the rest of our lives.

While one meaning of the word *sex* is "gender" (male or female), the word *sexuality* takes in *everything that makes a person masculine or feminine.* This "everything" includes all the traits, feelings, and values that combine to make you an individual and unique man or woman. Your sexuality is not something that begins during adolescence. Rather, it is an aspect of the entire person you are, developing and unfolding, like the petals of a blossom, throughout your life. From the moment of conception, we each grow physically, emotionally, psychologically, socially, morally, and spiritually. All such growth is also growth in one's sexuality; for it is as sexual persons that we grow.

It is surprising but true that in humans, the brain is the primary organ of sexuality, because the human brain is the source of sexual understanding and conscious choices. A person's sexuality influences *all* aspects of his or her conscious and subconscious thinking. A man, in a male body, has manly feelings and ideas. All of his human energies and attitudes are necessarily male. The same is true of a woman, in a female body.

Our sexuality is not merely a biological "function," like that of the lower animals. The human mind, enlightened by the human soul or spirit, can grasp the nature and meaning of a person's experiences. Because our minds are capable of making judgments, we can sort things out into such categories as "good" and "evil," "responsible" and "irresponsible," "true" and "false," and "ugly" and "attractive." The judgments we make have a great deal to do with our emotions or feelings, as well as with our intellect, memory, and will.

Figure 2.1 shows how the brain (hypothalamus), pituitary gland, and reproductive organs cooperate to bring about the changes of puberty, through the action of **sex hormones**.

You already know much about the human body and about the important role the brain plays in a person's life. What we would like to discuss here is what happens when people take a limited view of human sexuality.

In our culture, the word *sexuality* has for many persons come to mean little more than **genital activity**. Some persons take a still narrower view of sexuality and think of it only as "making babies." In either case, such persons tend to fear their fertility, and they are ignorant of the true meaning of

2.1 The Brain and Human Sexuality

The brain is the center of sexual attraction and has either a male or a female orientation in a male or a female body.

The hypothalamus tells the pituitary gland when it is time to begin secreting the larger amounts of hormones that will begin the changes of puberty.

Hormones secreted by the pituitary gland travel through the bloodstream to the sex glands (testicles in a man, ovaries in a woman). The sex glands in turn secrete their own hormones. The increase in the amount of the sex hormones at puberty causes a person to become fertile.

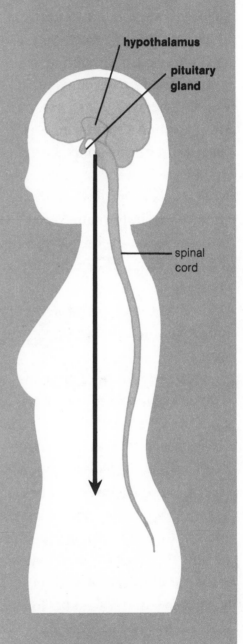

hypothalamus

pituitary gland

spinal cord

their sexuality. They tend to separate fertility, or their ability to have children, from their sexuality by taking steps to make themselves either temporarily or permanently sterile.

During adolescence, your body becomes fertile and mature; at the same time, your sexuality also matures. It is a natural, beautiful, and marvelous process. Medical science cannot even explain the whole process. But as our knowledge of human sexuality and fertility increases, we have to admire what nature accomplishes in us during adolescence.

Those of us who believe that the human body is as God wills it to be find it easy to see the human body as "fearfully and wonderfully made." And we therefore have no reason to fear our sexuality or our fertility. We do not shroud our sexuality in darkness or talk of it as if it were bad or evil. On the contrary, we accept our sexuality as natural and beautiful; we value it as God's plan for us; and we safeguard it because it is linked to the passing on of human life from parents to offspring.

Because you are a human being and not an animal, your sexuality is intimately a part of yourself. The person-you-are is a human being, either male or female, with an individual character shaped by your personality. How did you come to have that character? How did you learn to be a sexual person?

You were *born* with your sexuality; but your character has been formed and shaped over the years—mainly by your parents, in a family setting. You are a sexual person from the time of your conception, but you are learning to *understand* your sexuality with the help of your parents and other adults. You have seen adults live and love and work together. You have listened to your parents and other adults, and you have talked to them about all kinds of things. Your watching and listening and talking all had something to do with helping you understand your own sexuality, first as a boy or a girl, later as a man or a woman. The best way to "learn" one's sexuality is from loving parents, whose example teaches what words cannot teach. The self-gift of a man and a woman to each other in marriage is the best lesson any of us can give or receive in sexuality.

In your own family, you first learned intimacy, first learned to love and accept yourself and others, and first learned a sense of personal responsibility. By the time you entered adolescence, you had already received countless "lessons" in sexuality. Some of those lessons you no doubt rejected as not consistent with what you valued. During adolescence, as we said a few pages earlier, your sexuality as man or woman comes to the surface and announces itself through bodily changes that other people also notice. This is the period of your life when you establish your own identity as an adult, and when you begin to form new relationships with persons outside your own family. It is also the period when you will be called on, by a largely irreligious world, to accept a limited view of human sexuality.

Many adolescents nowadays have been persuaded that **sexual intercourse** is not something that belongs solely to marriage. They reduce their sexuality to genital sex. One result is a growing number of pregnancies among unmarried women, many of whom, fearing embarrassment or inconvenience, have their babies killed by **abortion**. Another result is an epidemic of **venereal diseases**, especially among young people. Those people who place little value on their fertility tend to abuse it. In fact, their fertility is something they would rather do without—at least for the present.

The presence of a large number of such people in society, who see in their sexuality only a source of pleasure, is an influence you cannot escape. There are several ways in which you can limit their influence—such as by the care you use in making friends—but the most important way is to *hold onto your own sense of self-worth*. We all know that it is hard to keep our self-respect if we do something that we know we should not do, or vice versa. Because we do not live in a consistent world, we need to be "true to ourselves," to what we **value**, and to our religious beliefs.

Because we believe that God is the Creator of all things, we believe that He is the author of human sexuality. And here we must make a clear distinction between the words *sexual* and *genital*. Because the brain is the most important *sexual* organ, we consider those things sexual which are seen as reflecting our total creative, intellectual, emotional, physical, and spiritual selves, as they are related to our *sexuality*. By *genital*, on the other hand, we refer specifically to the **genital organs** of reproduction. Hence we can say that the brain is a sexual organ without its being also genital.

Our sexuality includes genital organs for the sake of sexual intercourse. It includes sexual attractiveness between man and woman (for the brain recognizes the sexual attractiveness of another's personhood). It includes **fertility**, for the continuation of the human race. Because we believe that God is the author of human life, we believe that parents share with God the power of pro-creation, to bring new human life into existence. As Christians, we believe also that sexual intercourse belongs to marriage, both for the sake of the union of husband and wife and for the sake of their children. This, in a nutshell, is the reason why we do not abuse our sexuality.

Even apart from our religious beliefs, we can see that sexual intercourse is never an unimportant thing. Any selfish use of intercourse is clearly an abuse of another person. Human nature being what it is, sexual intercourse is a *natural* sign of a close personal relationship. When intercourse takes place between people who have no such relationship, it becomes trivialized; and they find it harder and harder to *have* a close relationship with *anyone*. For two human beings to have only a genital relationship is for them to act in a subhuman way. It often happens that persons who define their sexuality exclusively in terms of genital activity become psychologically bitter, withdrawn, nonsocial, and actually incapable of marriage. They train themselves to be unable to make a lasting commitment; they find it difficult to respect themselves, and they may become deeply depressed.

Sexuality is so profoundly a part of human nature that it must always remain a great mystery. None of us ever becomes fully mature, and none of us will ever fully understand our own sexuality. To some extent, we are each a mystery to ourselves, as well as to others. By coming to understand our fertility, we can better appreciate the mystery of our sexuality—and in that way appreciate also some of the mystery of God.

Christianity has always attempted to safeguard the mystery of human sexuality from abuse and distortion. It has guarded human sexuality and fertility with the virtues of modesty and chastity. It has held that respect for one's fertility and the fertility of others is closely connected with the respect one ought to have for human life, as something sacred. It therefore does not look upon human sexuality in a casual way; in fact, it encourages us to have a reverence for our bodies and to remember that God has designed them for us and has given them life.

Human Sexuality and the Reproductive Organs

To understand your own fertility, you need to understand your body's reproductive system. You may already have studied the human reproductive system in school, and we will speak here only about the more important aspects of this complicated subject. If you are reading about this subject for the first time, you may find it helpful to read this section carefully twice.

Of course, men and women do not share the same reproductive system. A man has male reproductive organs, and a woman has female reproductive organs. In the remainder of this chapter, we'll discuss each organ, explaining *what it is* (its **anatomy**) and *what it does* (its **physiology**). Then we'll conclude by explaining how the fertility of a man and a woman combine to bring a new human being into existence, through sexual union and **conception**. The illustrations show where the various organs are located and how they are related to each other.

Female Reproductive Organs

The **ovaries** are two almond-shaped sex glands, about the size of palm dates, located above and to either side of the **uterus**, or womb (*see Figure 2.2*). The ovaries produce **hormones** (see page 34) and contain thousands of **ova** (eggs). Three months after her conception, an unborn baby girl has about 400,000 immature eggs in her ovaries. Her ovaries store the immature eggs until the girl reaches the age of first menstruation. Then an egg is usually released at intervals of about four weeks*

---

* *The intervals vary from woman to woman; see Chapter 3, pages 32-33.*

2.2 A Woman's Reproductive Organs

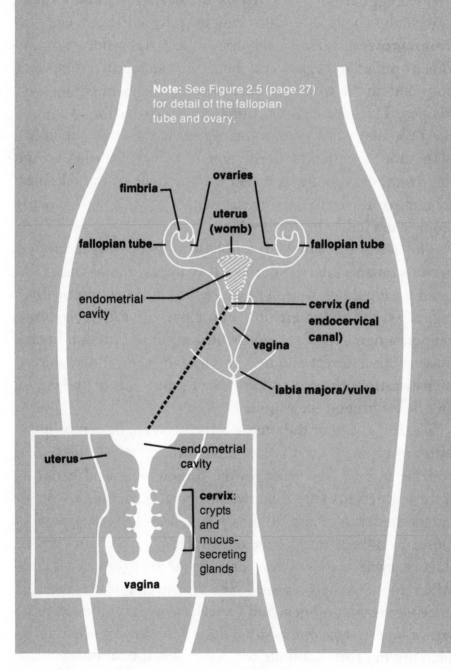

Note: See Figure 2.5 (page 27) for detail of the fallopian tube and ovary.

during the years when her reproductive system is active. The released eggs are not replaced by the ovaries; and in her lifetime, only about 400 eggs will be released. Each egg (or ovum) grows in a developing cyst (or **follicle**) inside an ovary. When puberty begins for her, the secretion of special hormones in the woman's body causes the egg-containing cyst to open. The release of the ovum is called **ovulation**.

At the time of ovulation, the egg is picked up by the **fallopian tube**. Slender tissue "fingers" (called **fimbria**) accept the ovum, and gentle, wavelike contractions of the fallopian tube move it toward the uterus, with the help of the microscopic hairs (**cilia**) lining the tube.

The uterus (or womb) is a hollow, muscular organ located in the woman's lower abdomen. It is about the size and shape of an upside-down pear. The uterus has a special internal lining, called the **endometrium**, whose purpose is to receive and support a new life. If an egg (ovum) is not fertilized, it breaks down within several hours. About two weeks later, during **menstruation**, the old endometrium passes out of the woman's body through the **vagina**.

The lower end of the uterus is the **cervix**. The cervix opens into the **vagina**, and it is the passageway between the vagina and the uterus. This passageway, the **endocervical canal**, is lined with **crypts** (tiny hollows or pockets). Before a woman enters the fertile phase of her cycle, her endocervical canal is closed by a thick mucus. The fertile phase of a woman's reproductive cycle begins a few days *before* ovulation, and ends when the egg decomposes. **Sex hormones** cause the endocervical canal to open, and the cells in the crypts *begin to secrete a slippery-type mucus* some three to seven days before ovulation; and they continue to secrete this special mucus until ovulation occurs. This slippery-type mucus forms hundreds of parallel channels which help **sperm** (see below) to move through the endocervical canal, in much the same way that a fish ladder enables fish to swim to a higher water-level (as at a dam). This mucus not only protects sperm on their way to the uterus and fallopian tubes but also nourishes them.

But this slippery mucus is present only during the fertile phase of a woman's "ovulation cycle." After the fertile phase passes, the cervical canal is again closed off by a thick mucus. The thick mucus thus acts as a safety valve: it is nature's way of preventing an aged sperm from fertilizing an aged ovum.

The **vagina** is the female organ of sexual intercourse. It is also the canal through which an infant passes at the time of

2.3 Changes in Cervical Mucus

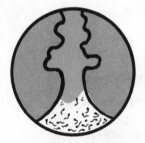 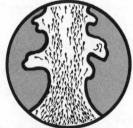 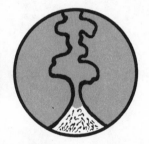

In the **early nonfertile phase** of a woman's reproductive cycle, the passageway from the vagina to the uterus is closed by **thick mucus**. Sperm are unable to pass through the cervix.

In the **fertile phase**, the passageway from the vagina to the uterus is open. A slippery-type mucus assists the movement of sperm through the cervix and nourishes the sperm.

After the fertile phase ends, the cervix is again closed off by a **thick-mucus plug**, blocking the cervical canal. Sperm are unable to pass through the cervix. This **late infertile phase** is followed by the **menstrual phase**.

2.4 A Man's Reproductive Organs

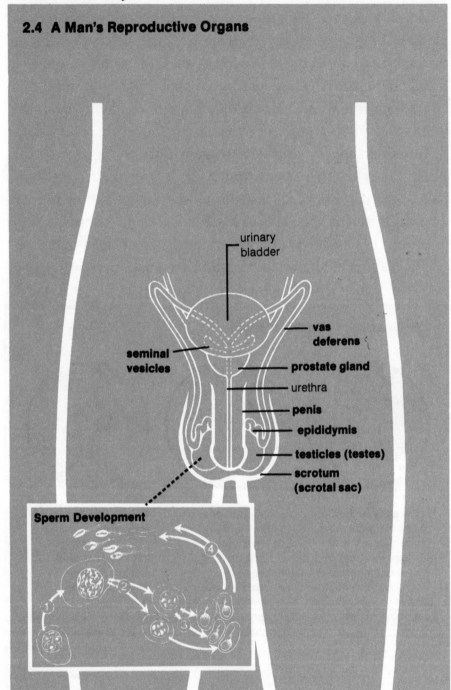

urinary
bladder

vas
deferens

seminal
vesicles

prostate gland

urethra

penis

epididymis

testicles (testes)

scrotum
(scrotal sac)

Sperm Development

birth. (The vagina stretches to many times its normal size during the birth of a child, and then returns to its usual size.) At the opening of the vagina are the **labia minora**, or inner lips. Where they come together above the opening into the vagina, they enclose the **clitoris**, a small organ that is extremely sensitive to stimulation. The larger, external lips of the vagina are the **labia majora**, which make up the larger part of the **vulva**. As we will explain later, on days when she is fertile, a woman can sense and recognize the presence of a lubricating mucus on the inner folds of the labia.

Male Reproductive Organs

The reproductive organs of men and women enable them to be parents. A man's reproductive organs, however, are quite different from those of a woman. (*See Figure 2.4.*)

The **testicles** are a man's sex glands. They produce male hormones and **sperm** (or spermatozoa). There are two testicles, carried in the scrotal sac just behind the **penis**, which is the male organ of sexual intercourse. The testicles are located "outside the body," so to speak, because they need to be at a lower-than-normal body temperature to produce sperm. Inside each testicle are thousands of tiny tubes lined with cells that will become sperm. It is estimated that during a man's reproductive life, beginning with puberty, the testicles produce trillions of sperm. (In the American number system, a trillion equals a million millions, or 1,000,000,000,000—which is beyond our imaginations' grasp.) As you might guess, each sperm is extremely small and cannot be seen except by microscope.

As sperm are formed, they are collected in the **epididymis**, which is a larger, winding tube that lies atop each testicle. The sperm mature in the epididymis. During sexual intercourse, the supply of sperm is ejaculated or thrust from the epididymis, through the ejaculatory duct and vas deferens, and through the **urethra** of the penis, into the vagina.

At the time of **ejaculation**, three other glands add special fluids or secretions to the sperm. The **prostate gland** is about the size of a chestnut and is located beneath the bladder. The urethra passes through the prostate gland; when sperm are ejaculated, the prostate gland adds a small quantity of a special, milky fluid that supports the life and assists the mobility of the sperm. The **seminal vesicles**, pouch-like glands that are connected by ducts to the **vas deferens**, also contribute a fluid containing nutrients for the sperm. The **Cowper's glands** are two pea-size organs, connected to the urethra just below the prostate gland. The combination of sperm and the secretions of those three glands is called **semen** (Latin, "seed") or seminal fluid.

In a woman's body, the urethra serves only as a passage for urine. Her urethra has its own opening between the lips of the vulva, separate from the vagina. In a man's body, the urethra serves both as the passage for urine and as the passage for seminal fluid during ejaculation. A man's urethra leads from the bladder and extends through the length of the penis. A special valve in his urethra makes it impossible for a man to urinate during sexual intercourse.

Conception and Implantation

The human reproductive systems of man and woman are obviously designed to lead to the conception of children. During sexual intercourse, the penis is inserted into the vagina, and ejaculation of semen occurs as a result of sexual excitement. If

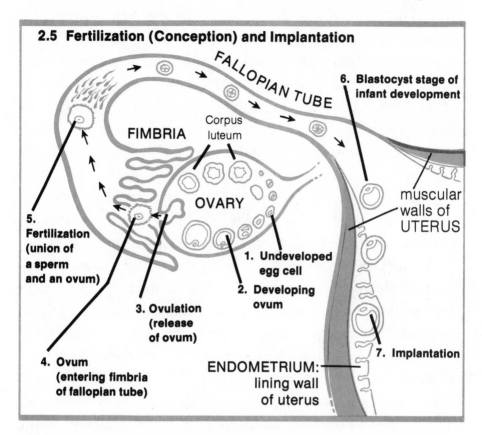

2.5 Fertilization (Conception) and Implantation

FALLOPIAN TUBE

FIMBRIA

Corpus luteum

6. **Blastocyst stage of infant development**

OVARY

muscular walls of UTERUS

5. **Fertilization (union of a sperm and an ovum)**

1. **Undeveloped egg cell**

2. **Developing ovum**

3. **Ovulation (release of ovum)**

4. **Ovum (entering fimbria of fallopian tube)**

ENDOMETRIUM: lining wall of uterus

7. **Implantation**

the woman is fertile and about to ovulate, there will soon be an egg or ovum in one of her fallopian tubes. If one of the millions of sperm released in an ejaculation reaches and unites with the ovum, conception takes place and a new human being begins his or her life. The union of ovum and sperm cells is also called **fertilization**. Fertilization usually takes place in the outer portion of a fallopian tube (*see Figure 2.5*).

Seven to nine days after fertilization, the new human life "implants" in (attaches to) the endometrium, the spongy lining of the uterus that has been prepared in advance. From the moment of conception or fertilization, a new human being exists, an equal combination of the **genes** from mother and father. The genes contained in the ovum and in the sperm that fertilizes it are the child's inheritance from previous generations. The child's genes make him or her a unique human being, with particular physical traits: blond or brunette, tall or short, brown-eyed or blue-eyed, and so forth. All such traits or characteristics belong to the child from the moment of conception, when he or she is but a one-celled person just barely large enough to be seen by the naked eye.

The child begins to grow as soon as fertilization occurs. During the first few days of life, the baby is nourished by his yolk sac while moving through the fallopian tube. After implantation, the endometrium lining the mother's uterus supplies the nourishment the child needs for the next few days of life, until the **placenta** takes over this function. The uterus, now filled with the baby, the placenta, and amniotic fluid, provides a safe environment in which the child can grow until he or she is ready for birth. Gradually, the infant in the womb goes through 41 generations of cell division, as eyes and ears and teeth and bones and skin and all the other elements of the child's body take on the form we recognize as a newborn baby. From birth till the end of adolescence, only 4 additional generations of cell division occur.

This brief sketch of our human reproductive systems hardly does justice to such a complicated subject. We hope that it at least gives you a better understanding of how closely connected our fertility is to our sexuality as male or female persons. In the next chapter, we'll talk about human fertility in more detail, and try to explain some little-understood aspects of the connection between fertility, sexual intercourse, and conception of children. □

CHAPTER THREE
Human Fertility

THE WORD *fertility* refers to the ability to become a parent. In a figurative sense, we speak of a "fertile mind," meaning a mind able to "give birth to" many ideas or insights. Similarly, "fertile soil" is land that readily nurtures and supports the growth of plant life. Our human fertility is our ability to become parents.

In specific terms, a person's fertility is his or her ability to supply a **germ cell** (sperm from a man, ovum from a woman) to the beginning of a new human being's life. Except for life itself, our fertility is our most valuable bodily gift. It is what enables us to become parents, and also enables each generation to pass the gift of life on to a new generation. The value of *human* fertility is hard to distinguish from the value of human life itself; because without the one, the other could not continue to exist.

Our fertility is hard to distinguish also from our sexuality. A man's fertility is part of his sexuality; a woman's fertility is part of her sexuality. Yet a man's fertility is much different from a woman's. Because a man is continuously fertile after the onset of puberty and a woman is fertile only for a relatively short time out of each cycle, a state of *combined* fertility exists only when she is fertile. (*See Figure 3.1.*)

In this chapter, we'll discuss some of the more technical aspects of those differences and help you understand and appreciate your own fertility. (We might mention here that some people are not fertile. When two people marry and discover that one or the other is sterile, they can be very distressed at their inability to have children of their own. In some cases, the sterility is temporary or is actually a case of "low" fertility and can be overcome. Sad to say, the most common cause of sterility in our culture is surgical sterilization —deliberately choosing to be made sterile by a surgical operation.)

The Signals of Fertility

Our fertility is dormant—sleeping—until our bodies enter the stage called **puberty**. With the onset of puberty, a young man's body becomes and remains *continuously fertile*. His testicles ordinarily continue to produce male sex hormones and

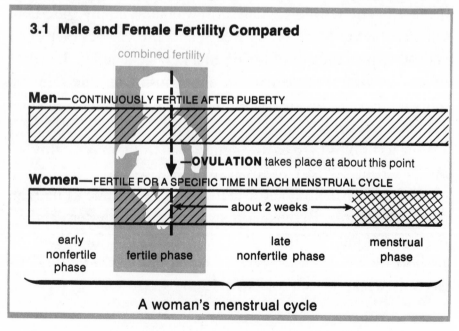

3.1 Male and Female Fertility Compared

combined fertility

Men—CONTINUOUSLY FERTILE AFTER PUBERTY

—OVULATION takes place at about this point

Women—FERTILE FOR A SPECIFIC TIME IN EACH MENSTRUAL CYCLE

about 2 weeks

early nonfertile phase | fertile phase | late nonfertile phase | menstrual phase

A woman's menstrual cycle

sperm for the rest of his natural life. The quantity of sperm produced is largest during the years of young manhood, and the "overflow" is commonly released during sleep in **nocturnal emissions** (or "wet dreams"). We have mentioned that spontaneous erections of the penis usually also occur frequently for several years following the beginning of puberty. The thought of a pretty girl or an erotic photograph or any of a number of other things can bring on an erection. This experience is something that young men need to accept as a fact of life and as a sign of their awakened fertility.

Sometimes a man may be unable to have an erection; this inability is called *impotence.* If impotence is the result of worry or exhaustion, it is a temporary condition; if it is the result of disease or injury, it may be a permanent condition. An impotent man is not able to have intercourse. We mention this point because **infertility** and **impotence** are commonly confused.

The important thing to know about a man's fertility, then, is that he is always fertile after his body enters puberty unless disease or some other cause brings about infertility. A woman's fertility likewise begins with puberty, but she experiences her fertility as part of a recurring process that has four phases. These phases are diagrammed in Figure 3.2; and you will probably find it helpful to examine that diagram before reading the next few paragraphs.

It is commonly supposed that a woman's menstrual cycle begins with **menstruation.** But actually her cycle *ends* with the shedding of the endometrium (lining of the uterus) during menstruation.

The first phase of a woman's cycle is the *early nonfertile phase.* When the lubricating cervical **mucus** begins to flow, she enters the *fertile phase* and usually remains fertile till after **ovulation**. The third phase is the *late nonfertile phase,* which, in turn, is followed by the *menstrual phase.*

Sometimes a woman may have a short cycle in which the *fertile phase* begins during menstruation, with cervical mucus also flowing then. There would be no *early nonfertile phase* in such a cycle.

The four phases of a woman's "cycle of fertility" may be summarized in this way:

EARLY NONFERTILE PHASE	VARIABLE LENGTH
FERTILE PHASE	SPECIFIC LENGTH FOR EACH WOMAN
LATE NONFERTILE PHASE	STABLE LENGTH
MENSTRUAL PHASE	SPECIFIC LENGTH FOR EACH WOMAN

As Figure 3.2 makes clear, the number of days from the onset of menstruation to ovulation can vary widely, whereas the number of days from ovulation to the *next* menstruation is quite constant or stable (averaging 12 to 16 days). A woman is *not fertile* during most of her cycle. Furthermore, a woman's cycle of fertility does not continue indefinitely, but gradually diminishes during her late forties; her ovaries release an ovum less frequently, and menstruation likewise does not occur as often. When menstruation stops altogether, she has entered **menopause**, a time in her life when her ovaries no longer release eggs in response to hormonal stimulation. It is not known why or how this happens.

We have used that word *hormones* without much explanation up to this point. This is a good time to take a closer look

3.2 The Menstrual Cycle

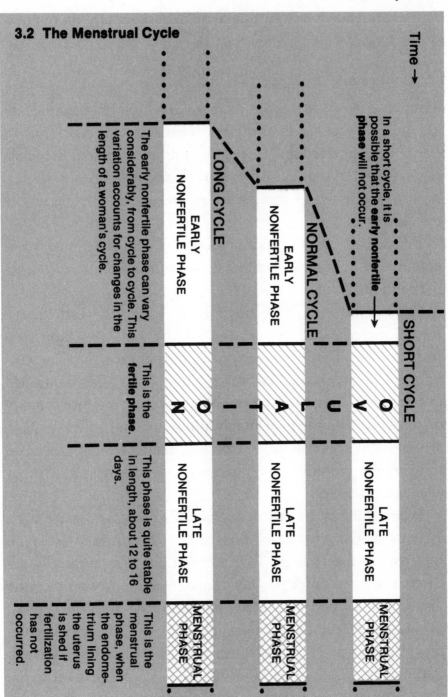

Time →

In a short cycle, it is possible that the **early nonfertile phase** will not occur. →

SHORT CYCLE
LATE NONFERTILE PHASE — MENSTRUAL PHASE

This is the menstrual phase, when the endometrium lining the uterus is shed if fertilization has not occurred.

NORMAL CYCLE
EARLY NONFERTILE PHASE — O V U L A T I O N (This is the **fertile phase.**) — LATE NONFERTILE PHASE — MENSTRUAL PHASE

This phase is quite stable in length, about 12 to 16 days.

LONG CYCLE
EARLY NONFERTILE PHASE — LATE NONFERTILE PHASE — MENSTRUAL PHASE

The early nonfertile phase can vary considerably, from cycle to cycle. This variation accounts for changes in the length of a woman's cycle.

at the influence hormones have on us—especially on our sexuality and fertility.

Hormones and Your Fertility

The word *hormone* comes from a Greek word meaning "to stir up" or "to set in motion." There are various kinds of hormones, secreted by various glands in our bodies, which regulate such things as bodily growth and metabolism. Puberty is a process set in motion by an increase in the *amount* of certain hormones.

Before puberty, all children, boys and girls alike, have small amounts of both male and female **sex hormones** circulating in their bloodstreams.

Puberty begins in the boy's body when his **testicles** (or testes) increase the production of the male sex hormone **testosterone**. This hormone causes further growth of his genitals and of the secondary "sex characteristics" we mentioned in Chapter 1—growth of facial hair, lowering of voice tonality or pitch, development of manly physique, and so forth. Men are usually taller and stronger than women because testosterone promotes the growth of longer bones and stronger skeletal muscles.

When puberty begins in a woman's body, the cause is an increase in the amount of the female sex hormone **estrogen** secreted by the ovaries. This hormone is what primarily accounts for the typical bodily characteristics of women—the distribution of body hair, the contour of the hips, the growth of the breasts, the completion of the growth of the reproductive organs, and so on. Estrogen tends to retard bone growth in the woman, just as testosterone tends to encourage it in the man. Consequently, women are generally not as tall as men.

Hormones travel in the bloodstream to stimulate actions and reactions throughout the body. We can notice their effects, but not their presence. The time when the sex hormones cause the reproductive system to begin to mature is called **puberty**.

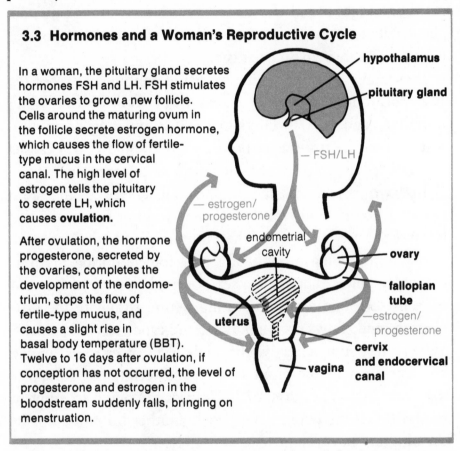

3.3 Hormones and a Woman's Reproductive Cycle

In a woman, the pituitary gland secretes hormones FSH and LH. FSH stimulates the ovaries to grow a new follicle. Cells around the maturing ovum in the follicle secrete estrogen hormone, which causes the flow of fertile-type mucus in the cervical canal. The high level of estrogen tells the pituitary to secrete LH, which causes **ovulation.**

After ovulation, the hormone progesterone, secreted by the ovaries, completes the development of the endometrium, stops the flow of fertile-type mucus, and causes a slight rise in basal body temperature (BBT). Twelve to 16 days after ovulation, if conception has not occurred, the level of progesterone and estrogen in the bloodstream suddenly falls, bringing on menstruation.

hypothalamus

pituitary gland

— FSH/LH

— estrogen/progesterone

endometrial cavity

ovary

fallopian tube

—estrogen/progesterone

uterus

cervix and endocervical canal

vagina

Puberty begins with a dramatic increase in the amount of male or female sex hormone circulating in the bloodstream. The **pituitary gland**, attached to the **hypothalamus** at the base of the brain, is the cause of the increased production of sex hormones. (*See Figure 3.3.*) The pituitary gland is often called the "master gland" of the body because all other hormone-secreting glands in the body take their instructions from the secretions of the pituitary. In some manner not fully understood, the pituitary gland is "nudged" by secretions from the hypothalamus into telling the sex-hormone glands that it is now time to step up production of sex hormones and get the changes of puberty under way. Clearly, if the pituitary gland fails to function properly, the hormone system of the body will be thrown off balance.

In a man's body, the pituitary gland continuously secretes two hormones, commonly called FSH (follicle-stimulating hormone) and ICSH (interstitial cell-stimulating hormone). FSH causes the testicles to produce **sperm**; and ICSH causes the testicles to produce the male hormone **testosterone**.

In a woman's body, the pituitary gland secretes the same two hormones, with much different results. In a woman's body, FSH hormone from the pituitary gland stimulates the ovary, encouraging growth of a new follicle during the pre-ovulatory phase. The female sex hormone **estrogen**, secreted by cells surrounding the maturing **ovum**, stimulate the production and flow of slippery fertile-type cervical mucus. When the ovum is ready, the high level of estrogen in the bloodstream tells the pituitary gland to secrete LH (luteinizing hormone). The surge of LH causes the ovum to erupt in **ovulation**. *If* the ovum is fertilized, another hormone signals the pituitary to continue to secrete LH.

If we may simplify the post-ovulatory phase somewhat, we will say only that the hormone **progesterone** (also secreted by the ovaries) then steps in to govern the following processes: it completes the development of the endometrium (lining of the uterus) in case the ovum is fertilized, so that the new life can be sustained; it stops the flow of the fertile-type mucus (*see* *page 22, and Chapter 6*); it causes a slight rise (about half a degree Fahrenheit) in body temperature; and it joins with estrogen in reducing the secretion of FSH until just before the cycle begins again. Some 12 to 16 days following ovulation, the amount of estrogen and progesterone in the woman's bloodstream suddenly falls if conception has not occurred, and this decrease brings on menstruation.

This explanation of how hormones regulate a woman's cycle of fertility is probably difficult to follow at first reading. It is sufficient if you understand that FSH and LH from the pituitary gland work together with estrogen and progesterone from the ovaries to cause the cycle. The sequence of phases in the cycle is the same for all women; but as we will explain in Chapter 6, each woman experiences a somewhat different *duration* for each of the four phases.

When a woman understands how hormones control the sequence of the phases of her cycle, she is better able to appreciate how those same hormones can affect her changing moods and mood-swings.

The fine-tuning and the precise interaction of reproductive hormones in a woman's body during her years of fertility are a marvel. So many events depend on so many other events that it is a wonder that pregnancy can occur. Yet it is possible for a woman to tell when she is fertile and when she is not by observing the signs and symptoms of her own fertility. This knowledge will help her to value her fertility and her womanhood. On practical grounds, many women have come to understand that the use of oral contraceptives to suppress any of their reproductive hormones does violence to their bodily ecology. Some oral contraceptives suppress the hormones FSH and LH, thus suppressing estrogen and progesterone.

Myths and Misconceptions

ABOUT WOMEN'S FERTILITY

• *Menstruation is the most important event in a woman's cycle of fertility.* Not true. The purpose of the cycle is to release an ovum from one of the ovaries; hence ovulation is the most important event in the cycle. In other words, it makes more sense to call it the "ovulatory cycle" than the "menstrual cycle."

• *Ovulation usually occurs 14 days* after *the beginning of the last menstruation.* Not true. Ovulation occurs 12 to 16 days *before* the *next* menstruation. The time between menstruation and the next ovulation is what varies and accounts for the differing lengths of women's cycles. The time between ovulation and the beginning of menstruation remains fairly constant.

• *Most women experience regular cycles.* Not true. The reproductive cycles of most women are irregular in their overall length. In a given year, the length of the cycle may vary by as many as 6 days, comparing each woman's shortest cycle with her longest.

• *If a woman does not ovulate and menstruate every month, something is wrong.* Not true. Some women may ovulate only two or four times per year. Such women are usually "subfertile." In the absence of disease, no treatment is needed. It is not good medical practice to treat these women with synthetic hormones "to bring on their periods."

• *The first day of menstruation is the first day of a woman's reproductive cycle.* Not true. Menstruation is actually the *end* of the cycle. But many women find it easier to keep a record of their cycles by counting that way.

• *The beginning of a pregnancy can be dated in relation to the beginning of the last previous menstruation.* Not true. This method is inaccurate at best. A woman can conceive a child only when she is ovulating—about two weeks before the *next* menstruation, which never occurs (a pregnant woman does not menstruate). An infant is likely to be born 266 days after conception, *not* "9 months" after the beginning of the mother's last previous menstruation.

• *Ovulation can occur more than once in a cycle.* Not true. Ovulation occurs only during the ovulatory phase of a woman's cycle. If in a given cycle more than one ovum is released, it happens within a 24-hour period, as part of the same ovulation.

• *Sexual intercourse can cause or bring about ovulation.* Not true. Mating causes ovulation in some animals (cats and rabbits, for example), but there is no evidence that intercourse causes it in women.

• *Women can get pregnant as a result of sexual intercourse any time during their cycle.* Not true. A woman of reproductive age can conceive a child only during those intermittent periods when she is fertile.

• *Contraceptives will always prevent pregnancy from occurring.*

Not true. No contraceptive is completely effective. The only sure way to avoid pregnancy is to abstain from genital contact. A contraceptive can "fail," of course, only when a woman is fertile.

• *A woman cannot become pregnant the first time she has sexual intercourse.* Not true! If a woman is fertile at the time of intercourse, conception can occur. It might *not* occur: see the next item.

• *If a woman has intercourse during the time she is fertile, she will become pregnant.* Not necessarily true. She is *most likely* to conceive a child under those circumstances, but it is always possible that she might not. (*See Chapter 6.*)

• *In order to become pregnant, a woman must go "all the way."* Not true. During genital excitement, a man with an erection may deposit a few little drops of seminal fluid without ejaculation; these droplets contain a very high concentration of sperm. If deposited on or about the vulva when fertile-type mucus is present, pregnancy can result even without penetration or ejaculation.

The result is that the uterus is unable to support the life of a newly conceived infant. Although oral contraceptives usually prevent ovulation from occurring, they can cause the abortion of a newly conceived infant by denying him or her a life-supporting environment.

A woman who uses oral contraceptives has no true cycles and no true menstrual periods, but only a bleeding that results when the taking of such contraceptives (and their artificial hormones) is interrupted or discontinued. □

CHAPTER FOUR

Reproductive Hygiene

IN THIS chapter, we are going to talk about the health of the body so far as fertility goes, primarily from a practical, medical point of view.

"Health" is what the word *hygiene* means; but *hygiene* includes the idea of *preserving* one's health. "Dental hygiene" deals with ways to preserve the health of the teeth and gums. Reproductive hygiene deals with ways to preserve the health of the reproductive system. Because men and women have different reproductive systems, some of the information in this chapter applies mainly to men and some mainly to women.

Cleanliness of the Genitals

A daily shower is the best way to keep your body clean. No one enjoys being near a smelly body! Good habits of personal cleanliness include cleansing of the **genitals**.

Boys need to keep their genitals—**penis** and **scrotum** —clean, and a daily shower suffices for this purpose. If a boy has an uncircumcised penis, he should pull the **foreskin** back from, and clean, the head of the penis each time he showers or bathes.

Girls likewise should take care to clean their external genitals—the lips of the **vulva**—when showering or bathing.

The **vagina** is a self-cleansing organ; "good" bacteria in the vagina act to keep it clean and in a slightly acid condition. Consequently—despite what numerous ads in women's magazines may imply—**douching** the vagina is rarely advisable. Frequent douching is likely to increase the chances of an infection in the vagina because it washes those "good" bacteria away. Girls are also well advised to avoid bubble-bath products, as another possible cause of irritation of the vagina. Irritation of the vagina can result also from the use of scented toilet tissue, certain laundry products (including anti-static products used in clothes dryers), and scented or deodorizing feminine-hygiene products (including sanitary napkins and tampons).

Sanitary napkins and tampons are absorbent pads to collect the menstrual flow. Napkins are convenient and simpler to use for young girls than tampons. Tampons have been linked to **toxic shock syndrome** (TSS), especially the type that manufacturers described as "super-absorbent." If such tampons were not changed often enough, the extra absorbency apparently drew normal moisture from surrounding tissue and caused irritation to the vaginal walls. The cells lining the vaginal walls were thus made unable to combat certain bacteria, which released toxins (poisons) that entered the body, causing high fever, nausea, vomiting, and shock—in some cases resulting in death. Such tampons are no longer for sale. Many women who do use (and change) tampons during the day, prefer to use sanitary napkins at night.

If a girl knows that one day she will menstruate, her first menstrual period (or **menarche**) will not frighten her. Instead, she can be prepared to take care of her needs herself. She will be excited to recognize in it a welcome sign of her approach to womanhood, and she will be proud and confident that she shares an experience all other women have had.

Probably the most common recurring fear among fertile women is that their next menstrual period will start before it is expected, or that the flow will stain clothing. A woman can learn to predict quite accurately when her next menstrual period will begin (*see Chapter 6*), based on her own pattern. If for some reason a woman does not ovulate during one of her cycles, her menstrual period may be delayed, and the flow will usually be different from her normal menstrual pattern.

Very frequently, girls experience cramping just before and during menstruation. A healthy diet, taking vitamins (especially B complex), keeping warm, and doing light exercise can improve this condition. Severe cramps can be alleviated by aspirin and use of a heating pad. If the cramps are serious enough to cause frequent absence from school or prevent participation in physical-education activities, a girl should see a doctor. Ordinarily, the fact that a girl is having her menstrual period is no reason for her to miss out on any of her activities.

When an adolescent girl goes to the doctor, the doctor is likely to need information about her reproductive system. These are some of the questions she will be asked:

Have you begun to menstruate yet? How old were you when you had your first menstrual period? How many days between the first day of one menstrual period and the first day of the next? Are your menstrual cycles usually the same length or not? How long do your menstrual periods generally last? How many tampons or sanitary napkins do you use in one day during menstruation? Do you ever have cramps or pass blood clots during your periods?

Because girls are more likely to experience genital infections than boys, we will mention some of the types of vaginal infections and their causes. The three most common vaginal infections are: **monilial vaginitis** (caused by a yeast or **fungus** organism); **trichomonas vaginitis** (caused by a protozoon); and **nonspecific vaginitis** (caused by bacteria other than **gonorrhea**; frequently caused by **clamydia**).

The symptoms of an infected vagina include one or more of the following: pain, itching, burning, stinging, unpleasant odor, or unusual discharge. Each case needs to be diagnosed and treated by a doctor.

The chances of developing *monilial vaginitis* are increased by douching, birth-control pills, antibiotics, and diabetes. Girls should use toilet tissue by wiping front to back, to prevent infectious organisms in the bowel from entering the vagina. Probably the most common cause of *repeated* vaginal infections is promiscuity ("sleeping around"—genital intercourse with various partners). If a woman develops *trichomonas vaginitis*, her husband also requires treatment; otherwise he may re-infect her after she has been treated, even though he has no symptoms.

Wearing cotton panties and vented pantyhose will help women to prevent infections of the vagina from developing. Panties or pantyhose made of synthetic material (such as nylon and dacron) hold body moisture near the vaginal opening, thus increasing the chances that disease organisms will enter the vagina and cause irritation or infection.

A woman is also subject to infections of the uterus and other organs of reproduction. "Pelvic infections" is a phrase that includes all such infections. They are common enough for every woman to take some commonsense steps to avoid them.

Much more serious than vaginal infections are the so-called venereal diseases.

Venereal Diseases

A venereal disease is a disease of the **genitals**. The vaginal infections we mentioned in the preceding paragraphs are not venereal diseases in the usual sense. A venereal disease is in most cases spread from one person to another by genital contact. That is, a person who has a venereal disease spreads it by any contact of his or her genitals with another's. The three most common types of venereal disease in the United States today are: **genital herpes** (or *herpes type II*); **gonorrhea**; and **syphilis**. All three are very contagious and are spread by genital contact; but *genital herpes* and *gonorrhea* may be spread in other ways too. Of the vaginal infections we mentioned earlier, *monilial vaginitis* and *trichomonas vaginitis* can also be spread from one person to another by genital contact; but these are not usually considered venereal diseases.

The word *venereal* comes from the name of the Roman goddess of love, Venus, who was associated with **erotic** love. Obviously, it is not a loving thing for a person who has a venereal disease to pass it on to another person; yet the spread of venereal disease has reached epidemic levels in many countries, including the United States.

Herpes type II (genital herpes) is a virus-caused disease that affects the genitals of men and women equally. It causes small blisters on the **penis** or **vulva**. The blisters break, weep, and merge as larger blisters. The pain caused by the disease can be severe. Before 1965, this disease was unknown, even though the virus that causes it is a relative of the virus that causes cold sores around the mouth. The disease seems to increase the risk of cancer of the cervix in women; and if a woman gives birth to a child when she is infected, the infant may be mentally retarded or may die. Though the symptoms of the disease seem to clear up after a time, the virus actually retreats into the body and eventually causes the symptoms to break out again and again. Because of widespread genital **promiscuity** in our culture, this disease is epidemic.

Except for the common cold, *gonorrhea* is now the most common infectious disease in the United States. The bacterium that causes this disease has developed into some varieties that are immune to treatment by antibiotic medicines. If the infection is treated in its early stage, the chances of a cure are fairly good. If not treated early or adequately, the disease can cause permanent sterility in both men and women. In women, the disease causes the **fallopian tubes** to become severely infected, inflamed, and finally blocked. Ninety percent of women catching this disease are unaware of any symptoms. A man who has intercourse with a woman who has *gonorrhea* usually develops drainage from the penis about five days afterward. In men, the disease causes a narrowing and scarring of the urethra. The disease is extremely contagious—so much so that it can be transmitted to female infants and children by contaminated clothing and bath water. The disease can cause blindness in an infant born of a mother whose vagina is contaminated. Doctors routinely treat the eyes of newborns with antibiotic ointment to prevent such blindness.

The third common venereal disease, *syphilis*, is less common than *gonorrhea* but has even more serious consequences. It is transmitted almost exclusively by genital contact, and its first symptom is a chancre or sore—usually located on or near the genitals. The sore shows up three or four weeks after infection. This disease is caused by a peculiar organism—a **spirochette**—that looks like a corkscrew when viewed through a microscope. If left untreated, the chancre will seem to clear up; but the spirochette actually remains in the body, invisibly, for many weeks or even years. A blood test can detect its presence in the body. In the second stage, the disease causes widespread eruptions on the skin and the mucus membranes, and inflammations of eyes, heart, and other organs of the body. In its third stage, *syphilis* causes tumor-growths and severe heart damage. If it attacks the optic nerve, it can cause blindness; and if it attacks the central nervous system, it can cause insanity. *Syphilis* is such a crippling disease that it can cause death. Penicillin is usually effective in treating the disease.

The widespread occurrence of venereal diseases is a serious public-health problem. They are a high price to pay for promiscuity, both for individuals and for society. Medical science has been unable to cope with the epidemic spread of those diseases, which tend to develop new strains resistant to new antibiotics, and whose symptoms often go unnoticed in early stages. Despite government efforts to warn against venereal diseases, the number of persons contracting them has continued to rise dramatically since the early 1960s.

We think young people should give serious thought to these matters. Recent statistics on the subject are sobering. What are the chances that a person willing to engage in sexual intercourse on a casual basis will be a carrier of one of the venereal diseases? (*Excellent.*) What are the chances that a person willing to engage in intercourse with a boyfriend or girlfriend or fiancé before marriage will already be, or will in that way become, infected? (*Good to very good.*) Even when considered only for their physical consequences, venereal diseases are clearly a penalty for abusing one's sexuality and fertility.

We do not intend to shock or frighten any reader with this information. We do strongly believe, however, that everyone has the right to be informed truthfully about these matters.

Fortunately, this national health problem should be of little concern to young people who resolve to save their powers of fertility for use in marriage, and to search out a marriage partner who has made a similar resolve.

How Stress Can Affect Your Fertility

In every person's life, there will come times of stress, times of physical or mental strain. Poor diet, insufficient sleep, monotony, and prolonged pain or illness can all cause *physical* stress. Fear, anger, frustration, and anxiety are some symptoms of *emotional* stress. Actually, we all derive some satisfaction from being able to cope with *some* amount of stress each day, because that coping requires us to use our creativity. Your ability to cope increases as you grow older; and your experience at coping successfully with little things helps you to cope with the big things that are likely to cause stress—things like a death in the family, unemployment, a relative who has become drug-addicted, a house fire, or an automobile collision.

Not that it is ever *easy* to cope with severe stress! Not at all. Coping with any kind of stress requires good judgment. The first step is to recognize the causes of physical or emotional stress that you experience. The next step is to "gather your wits about you" and decide how best to cope with that stress. In that way, you not only are looking after your health but also ensuring that you will continue to look ahead to the goals you wish to achieve.

The reason we are including this topic in a chapter on reproductive hygiene is that high levels of physical and emotional stress interfere with a person's fertility. The brain, being the primary sexual organ in the human body, reacts to stress and thus causes the whole body to be affected by stress. Anxieties about schoolwork, athletic competition, and disagreements with parents can interrupt a young person's fertility. Unmarried women who engage in genital activity cannot rely on the mucus symptom to avoid pregnancy; such activity *and its stress* distort the mucus symptom. Severe stress can suppress ovulation in a woman or cause **impotence** in a man.

Stress can also interfere with our thinking and decision-making. We may be inclined to escape from a stressful situation, or to "reward" ourselves for the suffering that the stress causes us. We might change our goals; we might abandon our sense of self-discipline. Some people react to stress by going off their diets or by going back to cigarette smoking. Young people may be inclined to escape their stress by seeking pleasure from genital activity, alcohol, or drugs.

Such genital activity often leaves young women with a new source of stress to cope with—pregnancy. The use of hallucinogenic drugs or alcoholic beverages in response to stress can lead to addiction and has many undesirable social consequences. Drugs ought to be administered to the human body only under medical supervision and for a sufficient reason. Many drugs increase stress and interfere with the hormones that affect fertility. Marijuana (or "pot"), for example, is far from being a harmless drug. It promotes feelings of alienation from friends and members of one's family; it decreases mental and physical proficiency, thus affecting one's abilities as a student or athlete; it leaves one with a feeling of inability to succeed, and thus encourages a sense of despair, which can end in irrational behavior, sometimes including suicide. Marijuana also tends to suppress fertility. To put oneself deliberately in a state of depression or paranoia is hardly the best goal one can have. A firm sense of self-respect and self-worth is the key to surmounting all forms of stress.

During the years when your body is maturing, you will be coping with all kinds of normal stress. From time to time, you may have difficulty coping with some of them. Patience, religious faith, and a sense of humor are your three most valuable weapons in the battle against excessive worry. The excitement of a football season or the tension you experience when preparing for exams are common examples of the kinds of stress that are coming your way. And you are probably finding that your parents, brothers and sisters, friends, and peers are either adding to or helping with that stress. Take the help when it comes, being aware that what is truly helpful is not always easy to recognize.

The times we live in tend to add to the causes of stress in our lives. Much depends on your own circumstances—such as where you live, what sort of friends you have, and what you expect of yourself. If, in our families, we all took the time to recognize and take into consideration each other's feelings, stress would be much less of a problem for all of us. It *is* possible to have disagreements within a family without resorting to verbal or physical abuse or violence. A "healthy home atmosphere" is one in which parents and children respect one another, are generous toward one another, and tell each other in some manner, "I'm glad you're alive and a member of my family."

Almost all of the lessons we get in coping with the ups and downs of our lives are lessons we learn in our families. The stresses of growing up and being a student or an athlete are relatively minor, compared to the stresses you may face as an adult, especially in marriage. Yet the ideal to aim at always is to make one's present family a place of peace and privacy and mutual support.

Finally, we would say a word about peer pressure, the influence that others your age are having on you day by day. In many ways, this influence can add to the amount of stress in your life. You may be in a situation where you sense that the important thing is for you to (a) own your own car, (b) find ways to drink beer without your parents' finding out, (c) get a girl or boy to "sleep" with you, (d) cheat on school examinations, (e) wear the very latest in fashions, (f) own all the recordings of the latest singing groups, and on and on. Such concerns can overwhelm young people so much that they become oblivious of the needs of other persons outside their circle of friends and even of other important aspects of life. This self-centeredness is psychologically unhealthy and very likely to lead to a selfish notion of one's sexuality.

Peer pressure is one of the ways in which young people especially are exploited by others who are trying to satisfy their own selfishness or insecurities. A bully is someone who thinks it is necessary to knock others down in order to feel important; there is a lot of bullying involved in peer pressure. Your choice of friends therefore has a great deal to do with the amount of stress in your life.

In the following chapter, we will talk about several other choices that face you as a maturing man or woman, all of them closely related to your sexuality. □

CHAPTER FIVE
Sexual Responsibility

WE HAVE looked at the *medical* consequences of promiscuity, and now we will discuss the *moral* consequences. As we intend that this book be helpful to young Christian people and their parents, we will speak frankly as Christians.

There is, in fact, little point in talking about "morality" apart from religious faith. Christian faith leads a person to look upon all aspects of human life in the light of that faith. That faith is the basis for *all* the important decisions that Christians make during their lives. Because sexuality is so much a part of what it is for us to be human beings, we are each faced with many opportunities to make decisions concerning our sexuality during our lifetime. In this chapter, therefore, we will be talking about the responsibility we all have, as Christians, for our personal sexuality. And we will approach that subject from the point of view of traditional Christian moral teachings.

Each of us has a responsibility to use our fertility in a manner consistent with our religious faith. We have, first, a responsibility to be *informed* about our fertility; second, we have a responsibility to have a *respect* for our fertility; and third, we have a responsibility for the *use* we make of our fertility. Furthermore, we have a responsibility not only for our own behavior in sexual matters, but also *for the consequences of our behavior.* We have a responsibility also toward other persons, to avoid any behavior that might lead them to violate their own sense of personal responsibility (or conscience).

It is hard to see how anyone living in our day can go through the period of adolescence without some inner turmoil, some temptation to "do what everyone else is doing," some tendency to get wrapped up in oneself, some feelings of rebellion against the authorities of one's childhood. Many psychologists think that our culture adds many potentially harmful pressures on adolescents; they think, for example, that many adolescents are pushed into dating before they are psychologically ready for it. Some parents of adolescents are guilty of urging them into patterns of socializing that are not necessarily good for their children's personality development. Other parents, on the other hand, offer their adolescent children too little guidance, thus letting peer pressure become the strongest influence on their children's lives.

It is very difficult, sometimes, for a young person to know whose counsel can be trusted. Nowadays, the voices of counsel and advice are numerous and often contradictory. This book is one source of counsel and advice for those who read it. We hope it offers safe counsel, good advice. We hope the parents of the young people who read this book will share our outlook and add their personal counsel to what we have included in these pages. And we hope also that the young people themselves will weigh the information and guidance we offer them, as they each chart a course, through more or less troubled waters, that will lead to personal independence and full self-responsibility.

It is possible that some readers of this book have already

made choices that are not consistent with the values we are attaching to human sexuality and fertility. They may feel uneasy about those choices, or have come to regret them. Our advice to them is to take a fresh start, to ground their decisions now on their basic beliefs and values. We are all free to reconsider our choices, *and* our values, and to change our behavior. That is the only way each of us can become the person we think we should be.

Feelings, Urges, Choices, and Decisions

As we mentioned in an earlier chapter, puberty or adolescence is a process over which you can have little control. The sex hormones start flowing, and bodily changes start to show. Your emotions also are affected by those hormones, because they affect your brain, which is the most important sexual organ in your body. They cause young men and women to become sexually attracted to each other—though girls tend to find boys interesting sooner than the other way around.

In animals, sexual instinct follows biological laws, which differ for various species. A female horse (mare) will mate with a male horse (stallion) only when she is fertile, or in heat; otherwise, neither is interested in mating. The same is true of all animals other than primates. In humans, sexual attraction between the sexes begins at the onset of puberty and continues more or less from then on. We humans differ from animals in our ability to make free decisions as to what we shall or shall not do. We differ in many other ways too, of course, because our minds are capable of thought. We can *know* and *judge* and *hope* and *laugh* and *be creative*; no animal can do such things. Of all earthly creatures, only humans are capable of spirituality, consciousness, and moral responsibility.

Animals never make decisions; we humans are always making decisions. Each day, your life presents you with many choices—what to eat for breakfast, what book to read, which friend to telephone, and so on. You make choices based on your *values* (that is, the principles you live by). Your values are based on such things as: your religious beliefs, your personal experience, your knowledge, and your hopes. Your religious beliefs lead you to place a very positive value on human life, and thus a very negative value on murder. You therefore protect and cherish human life and have a horror of murder. Your experience leads you to value one brand of toothpaste more than other brands. Your knowledge leads you to prefer one person's advice to another's. And your hopes lead you to place a high value on something (such as education) that will help you accomplish a goal you have set yourself (such as earning a living as a computer programmer).

In other words, we all live in a world in which values are everywhere. Values are involved in our decision-making all the time, whether it be a trivial choice (which type of dressing you prefer on your salad) or a very important one (whether to tell the truth as a witness at a trial).

Making *good* choices takes thought, experience, and foresight. When you were a small child, your parents made most choices for you. As you have grown older, more and more has been left to your decision. Your parents will continue to guide you, but eventually you will be on your own and will have to give reasons for the choices you make. You know you can't depend on your parents to continue to make important decisions for you; nor should you want them to; nor is that what *they* want. Instead, you have reached an age where you can be left to make many kinds of decisions for yourself. You have no doubt found that you have made a few mistakes—and maybe had to listen to a lecture on the subject from your parents.

As puberty works its changes in you, you will find yourself having to make decisions about new choices available to you. As your fertility and your sexual urge mature with the passing months and years of adolescence, you will sometimes find that your body is telling you one thing and your mind is telling you another. The sexual urge comes along at the same time that our reproductive organs are maturing. Our reproductive organs and our desire for sexual union exist in us because they are God's plan for the continuation of the human race. This desire varies in intensity from person to person, and from time to time. But it is a desire that we human beings *are meant to experience* as men and women. And it is a desire that requires us to make decisions.

In an ideal world, you could grow up as a happy member of a happy family, meet the boy or girl of your dreams at age 18, get married in an unforgettable wedding and honeymoon, begin earning good money doing work you love to do, become a parent to wonderful children who are cute, obedient, and intelligent, send them to first-rate schools, retire on a double pension, travel. . . . But ours is not an ideal world, so we settle for reasonable, realistic goals.

Marriage is not for everyone, of course; and no one should ever marry because of family pressures. But there is no doubt that men and women "are meant for each other" and that the sexual urge exists for the sake of marriage and the generation of offspring.

Let's consider next some of the choices that your awakening sexual maturity places in your hands, and the principles by which you make important decisions.

Moral Decisions Regarding Sexuality and Fertility

Just as all of our choices must be free choices (otherwise how are they called choices?), all of our decisions are moral decisions. That is, in themselves, they are either morally *good* or morally *evil*. What is true of decisions is true also of the acts that follow from them. To murder someone is morally evil; to *decide* to murder someone is also morally evil.

Christians have, in their faith, a powerful motive for wanting always to act in morally good ways. Numerous passages from the New Testament speak of the need to distinguish what is morally evil from what is morally good. Even the pagan philosophers agreed on the basic moral principles.

A given choice of action is morally good if it meets three conditions: First, *the action must be morally good in itself.* Second, *the motive or purpose for doing the act must be good.* And third, *the circumstances must not be such as to give an action an evil character.* All three conditions must be met by every free and responsible human act, or the act is evil. Whether you are aware of it or not, these are the principles you use to decide between what is good and what is evil.

Those principles are very abstract, of course, and not obviously helpful to us until we understand how they apply to our lives. Because we are making moral judgments about good and evil all the time, we should make an effort to judge rightly. Christians cannot *not* care about what is morally good.

It is true that a person may be led to choose to do a morally evil act out of ignorance or under the influence of a strong emotion. Ignorance or fear may lessen, or even eliminate, a person's responsibility and freedom. If we are to allow our reasoning ability to help us judge what is good and what is evil—as our Christian faith requires—then we need to educate ourselves, and our consciences, so that we can measure the morality of our conduct. We need also to form good moral habits so that we do not easily become slaves to our emotions. Self-respect is not possible apart from self-restraint.

In the preceding paragraphs, we do not pretend to have done more than review the basic principles by which we make moral decisions. Our main interest in this chapter is to help you make responsible decisions about your own sexuality and about your ability to become a parent.

We should begin by saying that your sexuality will always remain something of a mystery to yourself, and even more so to others. As young people go through adolescence, they are discovering something new about themselves almost daily. Their interest in themselves increases, as does their interest in members of the "opposite sex." But none of us ever fully understands the mystery of another person, not even of ourselves.

Traditional Christian moral teaching has always said that sexual intercourse and the physical intimacies that lead to it are morally good only within marriage. The love and commitment of husband and wife are the context in which children born of their sexual union are protected and reared. Sexual intercourse is God's chosen means by which human beings are to generate offspring. The sexual urge exists to lead a man and a woman to marry and found a family; and the physical pleasure that accompanies sexual intercourse exists to encourage their desire for physical union.

There is a tendency in our day to separate the physical pleasure that accompanies intercourse from the biological purpose of the reproductive system. This is a reflection of the ten-

Sexual Values Related to Chastity and Fertility Awareness

VALUES RELATED TO CHASTITY

• Building up your self-respect, self-worth, and dignity.

• Developing your sense of responsibility.

• Maintaining your freedom to be the person you wish to be.

• Keeping your personal integrity in your relationships with others.

• Knowing that you are not being used or abused.

• Being free from the pressure or the temptation to obtain an abortion.

• Being free from venereal disease.

• Being free from the side-effects of mechanical or chemical techniques of contraception.

• Reserving yourself for a lifetime commitment in marriage.

• Being respected as a person, not as a genital partner.

VALUES RELATED TO FERTILITY AWARENESS

• Increasing your self-knowledge.

• Increasing your self-confidence.

• Being better able to cope with the changes of adolescence.

• Being better able to look after the health of your reproductive system.

• Increasing your respect for your ability to become a parent.

• Being better able to cope with changes in mood or disposition caused by changes in your body's hormone system.

• Freeing yourself from exploitation by drug-manipulation of your reproductive system.

dency we have already mentioned—the tendency to separate "sex" from fertility, and sexual intercourse from its natural end.

The Christian idea of marriage is that it is a permanent, exclusive, and total commitment of a man and a woman to each other *and to their children*, and that human sexuality cannot be separated from that idea of marriage without losing sight of the purpose for which God made us sexual beings. Against this idea of marriage and of human sexuality stand those who favor such things as "trial" marriages, abortion, sterilization, and contraception.

The Christian idea of human sexuality is shaped by many things—by seeing that human fertility exists for **procreation**; by comparing the oneness of Christ and the Church; by seeing self-sacrifice as necessary to wholeness, holiness, and fidelity in marriage. Christians have a clear idea about what they are to become as sexual persons empowered with fertility. Christians have also a clear idea about what needs to be avoided if they are to achieve that goal.

Christians recognize that some things are an abuse of human sexuality and harmful to the human personality. Some acts involving human sexuality and fertility are clearly morally evil. The following actions in particular are not consistent with the traditional Christian idea of human sexuality:

- FORNICATION (sexual intercourse between those who are not married) is evil primarily because the circumstances are not consistent with the *meaning and purpose* of sexual intercourse.
- MASTURBATION (stimulating one's own genitals to achieve **orgasm** or genital pleasure) is evil because it reduces the

sexual power to self-love and turns it from its natural purpose.

- ADULTERY (sexual intercourse of a married person with
  someone other than his or her spouse) is evil because it
  gives to another person what was promised to one's
  spouse.
- CONTRACEPTION (the use of *artificial* means to prevent
  conception from occurring) is evil because it abuses and
  denies a unique, specialized natural process of the body,
  and power of the person—his or her fertility.
- STERILIZATION (sterility caused in humans by surgical or
  other means) is evil because it violates the integrity of the
  body by destroying *healthy* organs or tissue.
- ABORTION (directly causing the death of an unborn child at
  any stage of development) is evil for the same reason that
  deliberately killing any innocent human being is murder.
- RAPE (forcing another to submit to intercourse) is evil because it is a violent act against an innocent human being.

All of these abuses involving human sexuality or fertility are
evil either in themselves, or because the motive or intent is
evil, or because the circumstances give them an evil
character—or because of some combination of these reasons.

Without explaining in detail why Christianity has tradi-
tionally judged those abuses of sexuality to be morally evil, we
would like to point out that all of them also have consequences. Clearly, those who do not consider what the likely
consequences of their actions will be are not responsible persons. The consequences of evil may not be evil in themselves,
but they always interfere with the good order, freedom, or
happiness in people's lives. The adulterer attacks his or her

own marriage and often succeeds in destroying it. The fornicator often becomes a parent to a child for whom he or she is in no position to provide a stable family life. The consequences of abortion are death for the child and a weight of guilt for the mother. You may know of young people whose lives have been affected *for the worse* by the consequences of their own or others' behavior in sexual matters. The venereal diseases we mentioned in the previous chapter are not the only sources of human suffering as a result of sexual promiscuity or abuse.

Some young people decide to "try" sexual intercourse out of curiosity, and usually give no thought even to the short-term consequences of such behavior. Psychologists report that more and more young adults are sexually "burnt out" after years of promiscuity, and are unable to establish long-term relationships with others. Their sense of intimacy has been worn away by repeatedly abandoning old relationships—genital and otherwise. Young women are especially likely to think that they can use sex as a way of getting "love." They may think that genital activity establishes a "bond" between themselves and the men who seek such activity from them; the men, however, are generally seeking only a genital relationship, *without* any commitment. Misunderstanding about the meaning of the relationship soon causes it to disintegrate.

Romance, in other words, is not love—though it may lead to love. Romance (or infatuation) is based on emotions, feelings; love is based on knowledge, appreciation, and respect. Human bodies develop much more rapidly than human emotions do; and physical maturity is not a sufficient basis for a lasting relationship. The ability to keep oneself from being "carried away" by emotions is a mark of a mature person.

Much has been written about what "love" is. The Christian idea of love is very clear: it is an unconditional concern for the welfare of others, as of oneself. It involves a commitment to wish good for others, even those who are one's enemies. Love in this sense is a free decision to place the good of another on a par with, or even above, one's own good. This love results in self-sacrifice, not in reward or repayment.

At the same time, Christian love is not blind; it sees and admits faults, and works to correct them. It is concerned for both the spiritual and the material welfare—of oneself, of others. In Christian marriage, love includes mutual trust and respect. Our idea of love is strongly colored by our experience of it, in our families, with our friends. It is influenced also by the many kinds of *false* love that we meet with (for example, in some movies, television programs, and books). Young people understandably have a difficult time forming consistent values, with so many conflicting ideas of love to choose from.

We all need to know that we are loved. We need to touch those we love, and to be touched by them. Knowing that others do love us makes it easier for us to have the courage of our convictions, and to remain faithful to our values in the face of pressures to abandon them.

We might consider here some of the reasons why a young woman might be inclined to use *her ability to become pregnant* as a means of obtaining something she thinks she lacks in her life. She might seek to become pregnant simply to prove to herself that she is fertile and capable of motherhood. She might become pregnant in order to have some *leverage* in her relationship with the child's father (for example, to overcome the latter's resistance to marriage). She might use her pregnancy as a way to "establish" her maturity and independence in the eyes of her parents. She might be trying to escape from a life she finds hard to endure, or even to revenge herself against parents, relatives, and friends for real or imagined hurts. She might desire to have someone to love who will love her in return without question—her own baby. Or, finally, she may simply be craving attention.

We hardly need to say that these are all selfish reasons for any woman, married or unmarried, to wish to become pregnant. But they are the most common reasons why unmarried girls do become pregnant. And they suggest that many young girls are having a difficult time liking themselves and affirming themselves, their sexuality, or their fertility.

Both for practical and for moral reasons, an unmarried woman who becomes pregnant needs the support of her family and friends. The child growing within her womb is innocent human life; and steps need to be taken to ensure that the child is born into the care of a supporting, loving family. These steps include obtaining advice from the mother's pastor and from others whose advice is consistent with Christian charity and concern for the welfare of both mother and child.

Of course, *all* of us need the support of our families and friends. During adolescence especially, young people will find themselves becoming highly critical of their parents and other adults. This is a natural stage a young person goes through *on the way to becoming* an independent, adult person. Parents spend many years being patient with their children; adolescents can best return the favor at those moments when the faults and failings of their parents are most obvious. Some adolescents cut themselves off from their families *except* for those things they find useful or to their advantage—such as room and board, including free telephone! What most teenagers don't know is that their parents are actually far more interesting *persons* than they imagine.

If there is an ideal we could recommend, it is that parents and young people take an interest in each other *as persons*, as individuals living in *this* time and place, with interests and skills and hopes and dreams. Parents need to affirm their children; children need to affirm their parents. As children mature and learn to make their own way in the world, parents should encourage them to share in making the major decisions that affect the family.

As we stated at the beginning of this book, a loving family is the best school for education in sexuality. It is true that parents cannot share with their children their own experience of sexuality as husband and wife. Sexual intercourse is properly a private intimacy, and is debased by publicity (as by **pornography**). But the love between husband and wife does nevertheless teach their children what love is; for, by welcoming and nurturing the children who are the fruit of that love, they give their children the best possible education in sexuality, and in responsible use of their sexuality.

Sexual responsibility is really spiritual responsibility. We carry the burden of **original sin** throughout our lives; our will is weak and inclined toward evil. For Christians, education in sexuality aims to assist young adolescents by helping them appreciate the values of their sexuality and fertility and place those values under the protection of the virtue of chastity. Prayer—the lifting of the mind and heart to God—is an effective source of strength for remaining true to our values and commitments. To pray for such strength is to make a very important decision about the kind of person we each wish to be.

In the remaining chapter, we will discuss in more detail the cy-

cle of fertility that the adolescent woman begins to experience. We review the history of scientific study of this subject, and show how this knowledge enables a woman to be aware of the pattern of her own fertility. We will also discuss the Natural Family Planning method of using this knowledge to achieve or to avoid the conception of a child. This method is consistent with Christian beliefs about human sexuality and enhances the love between spouses. □

CHAPTER SIX
Natural Family Planning

WE HAVE mentioned in the earlier pages of this book many facts about human fertility that have only in recent decades been known to *be* facts. In this chapter, we'd like to look at some of the sources of our knowledge about human fertility, and show how this knowledge has become the basis of **natural family planning**.

Of course, we think it is important that *every* person be familiar with his or her fertility. Such knowledge helps a person to appreciate what a marvel of God's creation the human body is. But here we wish to explain how married couples can use this knowledge to *bring about* pregnancy, to *defer* pregnancy, or to *avoid* pregnancy. "Natural family planning" is the general name given to *natural* methods of accomplishing any of those purposes. The basic fact that makes natural family planning possible is not so much that a woman's fertility occurs in a cycle, as that *a woman can determine when she is in fact in the fertile phase of her cycle.*

Natural family planning is morally good if a married couple have a good reason to defer or avoid conceiving a child. It is possible for married couples to avoid having children for selfish reasons, and in that case their use of natural family planning (NFP) would be morally evil *for them*. It is even possible that a husband and wife might choose to use NFP in order to conceive a child *when their circumstances are such that they should not do so.* Natural family planning is an example of behavior that is neither good nor evil in itself, but is either morally good or morally evil for particular persons in particular circumstances.

How Fertility Awareness Has Grown

In earlier times, and still in our day, it has been common for people to have wrong ideas about their fertility and reproductive powers. One notion accepted widely during the early Middle Ages was that human life began as a *homunculus* ("little man") deposited during sexual intercourse inside the mother's body, where the child grew until becoming a baby. This idea prevailed until about 250 years ago, when a Dutch maker of microscopes, Antony van Leeuwenhoek (d. 1723), discovered the existence of **sperm**. The existence of the **ovum** was unknown until 1827, when Karl Ernst von Baer (d. 1876) discovered and described the process of **ovulation** in mammals. The next step was to understand that, in humans, the conception of a child occurred when an ovum and a sperm united—with each parent thus contributing half the **chromosomes** to the new human life.

In 1868, William Squire, a medical researcher, reported to the Obstetrical Society of London his findings that the ovulatory (or menstrual) cycle in women was the cause of changes in basal body temperature (*basal*, "at rest"—in other words, body temperature at the time of waking from sleep). Squire used this fact to record changes in the ovulatory cycles of women. Other investigators followed, confirming the accuracy of Squire's observations. In 1904, the fluctuations (rise and fall) of basal body temperature (BBT) in fertile women were shown to be related to ovulation. In 1935, a German priest, Wilhelm von Hildebrand, published a report showing how charting fluctuations in BBT could enable a woman to avoid conception. At that time, related attempts were being made to establish a woman's periods of fertility on the basis of calendar days (Calendar Rhythm Method; see below), but information based on fluctuations in BBT was an important improvement in identifying a useful sign.

New information came in the form of the discovery of the sex hormones (beginning in 1923, when Edgar Allen identified **estrogen**) and their functions. In 1928, two medical researchers working independently (Kyusaku Ogino, in Japan; Hermann Knaus, in Austria) published reports in which they showed that menstruation consistently *followed* ovulation by about two weeks, and that therefore the beginning of menstruation could be predicted if the date of ovulation was known. This information became the basis for the Calendar Rhythm Method of natural family planning. This method, often referred to simply as "Rhythm," is now obsolete.

Another important piece of information about cervical mucus lay unnoticed for nearly a century in W. T. Smith's book *The Pathology and Treatment of Leukorrhea* (1855). Smith observed the changes in cervical **mucus** and noted that at about the middle of the cycle (that is, at the time of ovulation) the mucus became clear and "stringy" in consistency. He correctly stated the connection between this mucus and a woman's ovulatory cycle. Others who studied this mucus symptom—a clear, stretchy, and slippery mucus—confirmed Smith's findings. But until the early 1950s, no one treated the special mucus as a **symptom** that women themselves could notice and understand.

In 1953, Dr. John J. Billings, of Melbourne, Australia, began his investigations of the various symptoms related to women's menstrual cycles, in order to determine why the Rhythm method was not as effective in practice as it seemed to be in theory. He came upon earlier researchers' descriptions of the cervical mucus and decided to question women about *their own* awareness of this recurring mucus symptom. Many women volunteered to cooperate in discovering distinct "rules" based on their own awareness of changes in the mucus at the opening of the **vagina**. The resulting rules were the basis of what is known as the Billings Method (or the Ovulation Method) of natural family planning.

Assisting the research into the mucus symptom were Dr. Lyn Billings (wife of Dr. John Billings), Dr. James B. Brown, and Dr. Henry Burger. Drs. Brown and Burger carried out laboratory studies of female sex hormones; they found that there is a definite connection between the time the mucus symptom occurs and the time of ovulation.

Speaking at a natural-family-planning conference held in Washington, D.C., in 1972, Dr. John Billings said information about the mucus symptom would be spread by women themselves, who would teach it to one another. By sharing information about the symptom throughout the world, he said, women could bring about the regulation of the birthrate by coming to understand their own patterns of fertility. The Ovulation Method is now being used in most countries of the world, and is winning ever wider acceptance. Many effectiveness studies have been made of the method, showing that it is about 99% effective among women who have been adequately instructed and who have observed the rules to avoid pregnancy.

The same is true of what is called the Sympto-Thermal Method, in which the information supplied by the mucus symptom is supplemented by observing changes in basal body temperature. There does not appear to be any measurable additional *method* effectiveness resulting from this added check.

This book cannot begin to give an adequate explanation of either the Ovulation Method or of the Sympto-Thermal Method of natural family planning. Because information about either method is still somewhat new and unfamiliar, we recommend that engaged and married couples receive instruction in either method from a certified instructor, rather than depending on printed information alone.

In short, more information about our reproductive systems has been discovered during the last fifty years than most people appreciate. This information has made us all more aware of the "ecology" of the various functions of our bodies. It has also given us reason for concern about the results of resorting to mechanical or chemical interference with the processes of our bodies. This concern underlies the growing interest in *natural* methods of family planning, as opposed to artificial contraceptives or sterilization techniques.

Advantages and Values of Natural Family Planning

Natural family planning is not medicine; it is not contraception; it does no violence to the reproductive system; it is consistent with human dignity; it is morally acceptable if a married couple make use of it with proper intentions; it does not look upon fertility as a disease to be "treated"; it "cooperates" with the natural processes of the human body; it costs

The Ideal Method of Family Planning

- It must be simple.

- It must be harmless.

- It must be reliable.

- It must be inexpensive to teach and to use.

- It must be acceptable in conscience to everyone.

- It must be able to be used successfully by anyone despite differences in intelligence, education, social conditions, and culture.

- It must be able to be used successfully during all conditions of a woman's reproductive life (such as during breastfeeding).

- It must be immediately reversible.

- It must not distort genital intercourse or involve any unhygienic or distasteful procedure.

- It must be able to be used by married couples to achieve, as well as to avoid, pregnancy.

no money; it does not deny our God-given "instinct" to become a parent; it does not contradict the married couples' human yearnings for loving and being loved; it places the "burden" of restraint equally on both husband and wife and encourages in them a willingness to sacrifice for each other's sake.

Now that we *do* understand human fertility, we can choose to live in harmony with it, or we can choose to bypass it, cancel it, or deny it. When husband and wife recognize that the other is willing to place sexual desire in second place and their welfare as a family in first place, they both interpret the sacrifices involved as evidence of the other's love. Natural family planning to avoid pregnancy requires of them that they refrain from genital contact during the times when the wife is in the fertile phase of her cycle. At such times, they demonstrate their love and affection for each other in nongenital ways.

People who think that human beings *ought* to be slaves to their sexual drive, and that satisfying their bodily appetites is what life is all about, will have much difficulty with natural family planning. We who are Christians do not believe that satisfying the body's "needs" is the purpose of our lives, and we see self-sacrifice as included in what it means to be a Christian. We believe that there are more important "goods" to be valued, and that our spiritual welfare is more important than our bodily welfare. Natural family planning is consistent with those beliefs.

In other words, the experience of married couples who have used natural-family-planning methods is that those methods preserve the dignity of sexual intercourse, encourage a respect for their fertility, and strengthen their sense of mutual trust and faith. They find also that they make the virtues of patience, self-control, cooperation, and generosity more important in *all* aspects of their marriage. And they become truly sexually mature human beings.

Recognizing the Symptoms of Fertility

Finally, we will summarize here the symptoms that accompany a woman's ovulatory cycle. (A man's fertility, once active, remains active, and has no symptoms as such.) And as you might suspect, the symptoms reveal just how complicated the reproductive process of a woman's body is.

The most specific and consistent symptom of a woman's fertility is the sensation of slipperiness or lubrication between the lips of the **vulva** before the time of ovulation. This sensation is produced by the slippery-type cervical mucus we described in previous chapters. It is quite different from the moisture that is otherwise lining the walls of the **vagina**. The sensation is similar to that which a woman experiences during **menstruation**.

Months before her first true menstrual period, in early puberty, a young girl begins to have an occasional discharge from the vagina. This discharge means that her reproductive organs are beginning to mature; but she pays little attention to it. Most girls, as they enter puberty, are more concerned about menstruation than about any less obvious discharge that no one discusses. The slippery sensation produced by the fertile-type cervical mucus usually *precedes* a girl's **menarche** (first menstruation).

It typically happens that, sometime following her menarche, a young woman sitting in a classroom suddenly experiences what seems to be the start of another menstruation. She is puzzled, because she had not expected her next menstruation for another two weeks at least. She excuses herself from the classroom and goes to the girls' restroom to check. She finds that her genitals are moist with a slippery fluid; she knows that this is not what happens at menstruation, but she does not know what is causing the moist and slippery mucus. Perhaps during the next couple of months she has a similar experience. She might begin to think that something is wrong; no one has ever spoken to her about it, or told her that this mucus forecasts her ovulation. She is likely to "teach" herself to ignore this symptom, and to focus her attention instead on the start of her next menstruation, which she does understand.

One of the purposes of this book is to inform adolescent women of this symptom so that they can learn to recognize it when it occurs. The slippery, lubricating sensation means that a woman is in the fertile phase of her reproductive cycle, that she is about to ovulate—and that she can expect her next menstruation about fourteen days later.

Furthermore, if she will mark a calendar with an X on the last day of the slippery, lubricative sensation and place a question mark on the calendar on the same day of the week two weeks later, she can see for herself that her next menstrual period will begin on the day of the question mark, or on the day before or the day after. In this way, she can predict the onset of her next menstruation and plan accordingly. (As we noted earlier, stress may cause a change in a woman's usual pattern.)

Most young women do not actually ovulate until they have menstruated a few times. Ovulation occurs on a more or less regular schedule only after a woman's ovulatory cycle is fully established. That process may take several years. The mucus symptom therefore can be expected to show up at quite irregular intervals at first, just as menstruation does.

A young woman should be familiar also with other symptoms and signs related to her cycle of fertility. These other symptoms are likely to vary or differ somewhat from person to person. One such symptom is a sensation of pain in the lower abdomen, on either the right or the left side, at the time when an ovary releases an ovum (that is, at **ovulation**). It is suspected that this pain (sometimes called *Mittelschmerz*, "middle pain") is probably caused by the rupture (breaking open) of the ovarian follicle from which the ovum is released. Some women may experience also a feeling of "tenderness" in their breasts, and perhaps some discomfort in the rectum, at the time of ovulation. Another signal that we have already mentioned is the rise in basal body temperature (about one-half degree Fahrenheit); this rise may occur any time from four days *before* ovulation to five days *after*, but usually occurs just after ovulation takes place. (*See Figure 6.1.*) Another sign—less common by far than the other indications we have

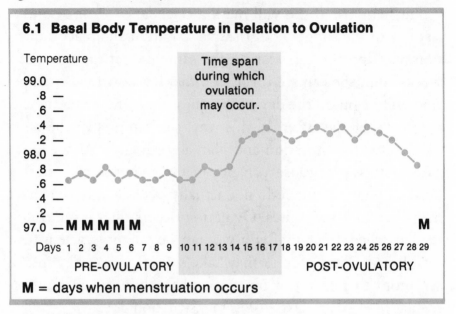

6.1 Basal Body Temperature in Relation to Ovulation

Temperature

Time span during which ovulation may occur.

99.0
.8
.6
.4
.2
98.0
.8
.6
.4
.2
97.0 — M M M M   M

Days 1 2 3 4 5 6 7 8 9 10 11 12 13 14 15 16 17 18 19 20 21 22 23 24 25 26 27 28 29

PRE-OVULATORY   POST-OVULATORY

M = days when menstruation occurs

mentioned—is slight bleeding (or "spotting") from the vagina around the time of ovulation.

On the following page, we show, in chart form, the sort of variations a woman can expect to experience in her cycle of fertility (*Figure 6.2*). As we mentioned in Chapter 3, such variations are normal.

Without question, the *key* to the understanding of human fertility is the significance of the cervical mucus and how it functions. Without question also, something so profoundly a part of human nature as sexuality must remain a great mystery. An understanding of our fertility is a window through which we can see the mystery of our sexuality, while marveling at the One whose goodness has authored it. □

6.2 Interrelationships of a Woman's Reproductive Cycle

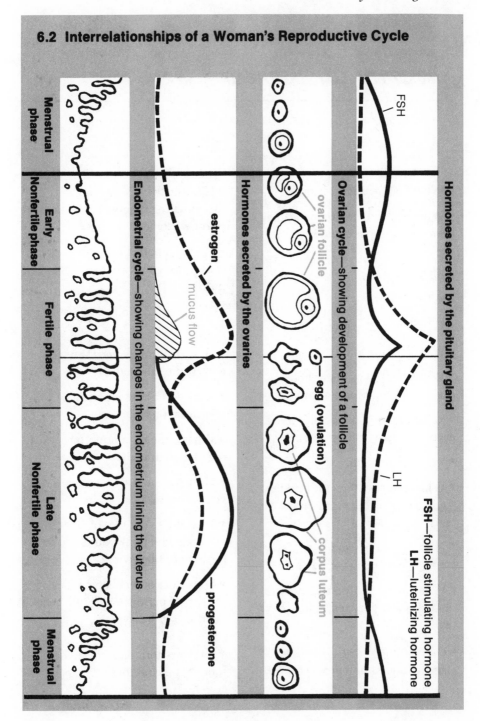

Menstrual phase | Early Nonfertile phase | Fertile phase | Late Nonfertile phase | Menstrual phase

Endometrial cycle—showing changes in the endometrium lining the uterus

Hormones secreted by the ovaries

estrogen

mucus flow

progesterone

Ovarian cycle—showing development of a follicle

ovarian follicle

egg (ovulation)

corpus luteum

Hormones secreted by the pituitary gland

FSH

LH

FSH—follicle stimulating hormone
LH—luteinizing hormone

Questions for Review

- What does *sexuality* mean?

- What is the difference in meaning between *sex* and *sexuality*?

- What is the difference between *sexual* and *genital*?

- What is fertility?

- What is menstruation?

- What is ovulation?

- What organs in a man's body enable him to become a parent?

- What organs in a woman's body enable her to become a parent?

- What is the uterus?

- What influence does the pituitary gland have on your reproductive system?

- How are ovaries and testicles similar, and how are they different?

- What are sex hormones, and how do they affect your reproductive system?

- Do men and women share any identical organs of reproduction?

- Is it true that a woman who is menstruating cannot play basketball or other strenuous games?

- What is another name for the canal through which infants are born?

- How can a person know whether he or she is fertile?

- What is the difference between adolescence and puberty?

- Why don't boys experience menstruation?

- What is the most important sexual organ in your body?

- How do your values influence your behavior?

- How does your idea of what sort of person you think you *should* be influence your behavior?

- How does other people's idea of the sort of person you should be influence your behavior?

- How do hormones affect your moods and emotions?

• Can you give the ordinary names for the reproductive organs of both a man's body and a woman's body?

• Do you understand your own system of fertility well enough to explain it to others your age?

• Is it true that a woman can become pregnant anytime after she enters puberty?

• What is menopause?

• Can you name any abuses of human fertility and explain why they *are* abuses?

• What is the difference between infertility and sterility?

• What is the difference between infertility and impotence?

• What is circumcision?

• What causes men to be generally taller than women?

• Do boys and girls usually enter puberty at about the same age?

• What is *natural* family planning?

• What is the menstrual cycle?

• How can a woman predict within a day or so when her next menstruation will begin?

• What is sexual intercourse?

• What are venereal diseases?

• What is the best way to prevent the spread of venereal diseases?

• What is the difference between a vaginal infection and a venereal disease?

• Can you identify ways in which others your age are adding to the stress in your life?

• How do adolescents differ from adults, generally speaking?

• What is chastity?

• What are the practical advantages of living chastely?

• What are the practical advantages of your understanding the fertility of both men and women?

Further Reading

For younger adolescents:

Vincenza Gagliostro, S.S.N.D., *Am I OK If I Feel the Way I Do?* (New York: Doubleday, 1981). Softcover. A good discussion of feelings and emotions in relation to religious faith.

James A. Dobson, *Preparing for Adolescence* (Santa Ana, Calif.: Vision House, 1978). Softcover. Sound information about the problems that young people typically face during adolescence.

Lennart Nilsson, *A Child Is Born,* rev. ed. (New York: Delacorte, 1977). Hardcover. A beautifully illustrated book for family reference.

John Powell, S.J., *Why Am I Afraid to Tell You Who I Am?* (Niles, Ill.: Argus Communications, 1969). Softcover. An insightful book on self-awareness, dealing with emotions, courage, and mature love.

John H. McGoey, *Sex, Love, and the Believing Boy,* and *Sex, Love, and the Believing Girl* (Scarborough, Ontario: The Book Department, 1980). Softcover. These two books help young people to sort out the rights and wrongs of sexual versus genital relationships. Available from The Book Department, 2685 Kingston Road, Scarborough, Ontario, Canada M1M 1M4. Price of each title: $3.00.

For older adolescents:

Walter Trobisch, *Living with Unfulfilled Desires* (Downers Grove, Ill.: InterVarsity Press). Softcover. A practical book, for adolescents and their parents.

John Powell, S.J., *Unconditional Love* (Niles, Ill.: Argus Communications, 1978). Softcover. Presents unconditional love as the only kind of love that deserves the name.

Donald DeMarco, *Sex and the Illusion of Freedom* (Toronto: Mission Press, 1981). Softcover. Shows the true face of what is falsely called "love" and "freedom."

Mary R. Joyce, *How Can a Man and a Woman Be Friends?* (Collegeville, Minn.: Liturgical Press). Pamphlet. Explains how a person-centered (as opposed to a genital-centered) sexuality frees a couple for equality and friendship.

Conrad W. Baars, *Born Only Once: The Miracle of Affirmation* (Chicago: Franciscan Herald Press, 1975). Softcover. A helpful discussion of the importance of self-affirmation to one's happiness.

For engaged and married couples:

John and Nancy Ball, *Joy in Human Sexuality* (Collegeville, Minn.: Liturgical Press). Pamphlet. Discusses the *meaning* of natural family planning and the positive benefits of periodic abstinence.

Evelyn Billings and Ann Westmore, *The Billings Method: Controlling Fertility without Drugs or Devices* (New York: Random House, 1980). Hardcover. A delightfully readable book discussing all aspects of the Billings Method of natural family planning.

John J. Billings, *The Ovulation Method of Natural Family Planning*, rev. ed. (Collegeville, Minn.: Liturgical Press, 1973). Softcover. A simple, concise, but thorough explanation of the Ovulation Method, by its originator.

Henry V. Sattler, C.SS.R., *Sex Is Alive and Well and Flourishing among Christians* (Huntington, Ind.: Our Sunday Visitor, Inc., 1980). Softcover. About the role that sex should play in our lives.

Terrie Guay, *The Personal Fertility Guide: How to Avoid or Achieve Pregnancy Naturally* (New York: Putnam, 1980). Softcover. A presentation of the advantages of the Ovulation Method of natural family planning, laced generously with valuable information on the holistic-medicine approach to health.

Robert Joyce, *Human Sexual Ecology* (University Press of America, 1981). Softcover. An examination of human sexuality, presenting the Judeo-Christian ethic from an unusual perspective.

Gerald Weiss, *On Becoming Married: The Art of a Loving Marriage* (Huntington, Ind.: Our Sunday Visitor, Inc., 1982). Softcover. Explains how intimacy and sexuality are gradually incorporated into marriages.

Glossary

Abortifacient: a substance or device that causes **abortion**, before or after **implantation**.

Abortion: direct destruction of the life of an unborn child at any stage of development following **conception**.

Adolescence: in human life, the period between the awakening of one's fertility (**puberty**) and physical maturity or adulthood.

Adoption: taking on the legal responsibility of rearing another's child as one's own.

Adultery: voluntary sexual intercourse between a married person and one who is not the spouse.

Amenorrhea: prolonged absence of **menstruation**.

Anatomy, human: study of the physical structures of the body and their relationships.

Anovulatory: "without ovulation"; a menstrual cycle in which ovulation does not occur is an anovulatory cycle.

Bacteria: single-celled micro-organisms: some cause disease, some protect against disease-causing organisms.

Basal body temperature: the temperature of the human body at rest, unaffected by activity.

Billings Method: see Ovulation Method.

Birth control: see Contraception.

Blastocyst: a stage in human development, occurring 7 to 9 days after **conception**; consists of an outer layer that forms the **placenta**, and an inner pole from which the baby's body develops. See **Embryo**, **Zygote**.

Calendar Rhythm: an early, now obsolete form of **natural family planning**, by which the length of a woman's previous cycles was used to determine the fertile phase of subsequent cycles.

Cervical mucus: see Mucus.

Cervix: the lower, narrow part (or neck) of the **uterus**.

Chromosome: one of the rod-like bodies of a cell nucleus that contains **genes**. There are 46 chromosomes in a human cell, 23 in each **germ cell**.

Circumcision: surgical removal of a portion of the **foreskin** from the **penis**.

Clamydia: an unusual micro-organism that causes genital infections in women.

Climacteric: see **Menopause**.

Coitus: a name for genital intercourse. See **Sexual intercourse**.

Conceive: become pregnant. See **Conception**, **Pregnancy**.

Conception: beginning of a new human life when a **sperm** and an **ovum** unite; the moment when **pregnancy** begins; fertilization.

Contraception: use of mechanical devices or chemical substances to prevent the union of **sperm** and **ovum**.

Corpus luteum: the "yellow body" or structure that forms from the ruptured ovarian **follicle**; it produces both **estrogen** and **progesterone** after **ovulation**.

Cowper's glands: pea-sized glands that empty into the male **urethra**, contributing to **semen**.

Crypt: a small cavity.

Cycle: a series of events that recurs with some regularity.

Cyst: a sac-like structure in the body.

Douche: a stream of water or other solution directed into the **vagina** to wash it out.

Ecology: the pattern of relationships between living things and their environments.

Ejaculation: the forceful ejection of **semen** from the **penis**.

Embryo: an early stage in the development of a baby, from the second to the eighth week of life. See **Blastocyst**, **Fetus**, **Zygote**.

Endocervical canal: passageway between the lower part of the **uterus** and the **vagina**; the lining of the cervix where the mucus-secreting glands are located.

Endometrium: the inner lining of the **uterus**; during each cycle it prepares for **pregnancy**, and it is shed in **menstruation** if pregnancy does not occur.

Epidemic: outbreak of a disease that spreads readily and rapidly.

Epididymis: the tube that carries **sperm** from the **testes** to the **vas deferens**. See page 24.

Erotic: anything that arouses sexual desire.

Estrogen: the ovarian **hormone** that causes production of the fertile-type cervical **mucus** and development of secondary sex-characteristics (see page 10) in women.

Fallopian tube: in women, one of two tube-like structures opening from the side of the **uterus**, extending toward an **ovary**; **ova**, **sperm**, and **blastocysts** move through it. See page 21.

Fertility: the ability to become a parent, to transmit one's own life.

Fertilization: see **Conception**.

Fetus: a baby from the eighth week of development till birth.

Fimbria: delicate tissue-fingers at the outer end of a **fallopian tube**.

Follicle: a tiny sac-like structure; in an **ovary**, the **cyst** where an **ovum** develops.

Foreskin: loose skin that covers the head of the penis; the foreskin is often removed by **circumcision**.

Fornication: genital intercourse between unmarried persons.

FSH: follicle-stimulating hormone; a hormone secreted by the **pituitary gland**, causing the development of ova (see **Ovum**) in women and **sperm** in men.

Fungus: a primitive life-form that multiplies by a nonsexual, budding process; a cause of **vaginitis**.

Gene: the basic unit of **heredity**, carried by **chromosomes**.

Genital activity: behavior involving the **genital organs**.

Genital Herpes (Herpes type II): a viral infection that attacks the genital organs of both men and women, causing distressfully painful blisters.

Genital organs (genitals): in a general sense, the reproductive organs; more commonly, the external reproductive organs (**vulva**, **clitoris**, and **vagina** in women; **penis**, **testicles**, and **scrotum** in men).

Genital relations: interaction of two persons involving the **genital organs**.

Germ cell: cell of biological reproduction; **sperm** from men, **ovum** from women.

Gonad: a sex gland; the **ovary** in the female, the **testicle** in the male.

Gonorrhea: a highly contagious venereal disease transmitted by genital intercourse; can result in **sterility**; caused by the bacterium "Neisseria gonorrhea."

Heat: in animals other than primates, a state in which the female will accept mating with a male; this state occurs strictly under the control of hormones.

Heredity: the physical characteristics passed on from parents to offspring.

Herpes type II: see **Genital Herpes**.

Hormone: a complex chemical substance produced by a gland and carried by the bloodstream to influence other organs or body parts.

Hypothalamus: a major "control center" of the body, located at the base of the brain, above the **pituitary gland**, with which it interacts.

ICSH: interstitial cell-stimulating hormone; a hormone secreted by the pituitary gland in men, stimulating production of **testosterone** by the **testicles**. Identical to **LH** in women.

Implantation: imbedding of the **blastocyst** in the **endometrium**.

Impotence: in men, an inability to achieve or maintain erection of the penis, hence an inability to accomplish intercourse.

Infertility: inability to become a parent; women are naturally infertile during their menstrual cycles except for the ovulatory phase. See pages 30, 78-79.

Intercourse: see **Sexual intercourse**.

Labia majora: outer lips of the **vulva**.

Labia minora: inner lips of the **vulva**.

LH: luteinizing hormone; secreted by the **pituitary gland** in women, triggering **ovulation** and the formation of the **corpus luteum**. Identical to **ICSH** in men.

Masturbation: stimulating one's own genitals to achieve **orgasm** or sexual pleasure.

Menarche: a woman's first **menstruation**; usually occurs between ages 10 and 17.

Menopause (climacteric): the time in a woman's life when she ceases to experience **menstruation**.

Menses: see **Menstruation**.

Menstrual cycle (ovulatory cycle): in women, the reproductive cycle, commonly measured as the time interval from the beginning of one **menstruation** to the beginning of the next.

Menstruation (menses; period): the shedding of the **endometrium** about 12 to 16 days after **ovulation** if pregnancy does not occur; the last phase of a woman's **menstrual cycle**.

Miscarriage: a pregnancy that ends prematurely through some natural cause. Compare **Abortion**.

Mittelschmertz: lower abdominal pain associated with **ovulation** (page 75).

Monilial vaginitis: vaginal infection caused by a yeast or **fungus** organism called "Candida albicana."

Mucus, cervical: a slippery, lubricative substance produced by glands of the **endocervical canal** under the influence of **estrogen** during the ovulatory (fertile) phase of a woman's cycle; this mucus prolongs **sperm** life and aids them in achieving **conception**.

Natural family planning (NFP): methods of achieving or avoiding pregnancy based on knowledge of the **signs** and **symptoms** of human **fertility**; requires abstinence from genital contact during the ovulatory (fertile) phase of a woman's cycle to avoid pregnancy. See Chapter 6.

Nocturnal emission (wet dream): in men, periodic release of **semen** during sleep.

Nonspecific vaginitis: vaginal infection caused by an organism other than that which causes **gonorrhea**; frequently caused by **clamydia**.

Orgasm: in men and women, pleasurable climax of genital stimulation; in men, accompanied by **ejaculation**.

Original sin: the Christian doctrine that the sin of Adam (Genesis 2.8-3.24) is passed on to all human beings as a state of privation of grace and weakening of human nature and natural human powers.

Ovarian follicle: see **Follicle**.

Ovaries: female sex glands, in which ova (eggs) are brought to maturity. See **Ovulation**; **Ovum**.

Ovulation: release of a mature **ovum** by an ovarian follicle during the ovulatory phase of a woman's **menstrual cycle**.

Ovulation Method (Billings Method): a method of **natural family planning** developed by Drs. John and Evelyn Billing, based on the **mucus** symptom as signaling the fertile phase of a woman's **menstrual cycle**.

Ovulatory cycle: see **Menstrual cycle**.

Ovum, pl. **ova**: egg(s); female germ cell, produced by the ovaries; one mature ovum is usually released by one of the ovaries during the ovulatory (fertile) phase of a woman's cycle. See **Conception**.

Pelvic Inflammatory Disease (PID): infection of a woman's internal pelvic reproductive organs; can cause sterility.

Penis: one of the male **genital organs**. See **Sexual intercourse**, and page 24.

Period, menstrual: see **Menstruation**.

Physiology, human: study of the functions and activities of bodily organs.

Pituitary gland: master hormonal gland of the human body, located at the base of the brain.

Placenta: the organ that forms from the **blastocyst** and attaches to the **endometrium** during an early stage of pregnancy; it nourishes the developing baby.

Pornography: in general, any deliberate attempt to arouse **erotic** feelings as an end in themselves.

Pregnancy: the period between **conception** and birth.

Progesterone: female sex hormone secreted by the **corpus luteum** after ovulation; prepares the **endometrium** for **implantation** by a fertilized ovum (**blastocyst**); stops the flow of cervical **mucus** by opposing the influence of **estrogen**.

Promiscuity, genital: the practice of engaging in genital relations with different partners.

Prostate gland: an organ that surrounds the neck of the bladder and the **urethra** in the male; contributes most of the fluid volume of **semen**.

Puberty: the time when one first becomes fertile. See **Adolescence**.

Rape: forcing another person to submit to genital intercourse.

Reproduction, human: the process by which new human life is generated.

Rhythm Method: see **Calendar Rhythm**.

Scrotum: in men, external pouch suspended behind the base of the penis, containing the **testicles**. See page 24.

Semen (seminal fluid): **sperm** combined with secretions of the **prostate gland, cowper's glands**, and **seminal vesicles**.

Seminal vesicles: in men, reproductive organs that secrete a thick fluid that makes up part of the **semen**.

Sensualism: believing that, or behaving as if, physical pleasure and self-gratification are the main purposes of human life.

Sex hormones: those hormones secreted by the reproductive glands of the body.

Sexploitation: a term referring to abuse of human sexuality for personal, economic, or political gain.

Sexual intercourse: as used in this book, the bodily union of man and woman in marriage, as a sign of their mutual love and commitment; also, this union as accomplished by insertion of the erect **penis** in the **vagina**, culminating in **orgasm** and ejaculation of **semen**.

Sexuality, human: the sum of the physical, mental, emotional, and spiritual traits and values that make up an individual male or female person.

Sexually transmitted disease (STD): see **Venereal disease**.

Sign, physiological: an observable or measurable manifestation of some bodily process (e.g., blood pressure).

Sperm (spermatozoa): male germ cells, produced by the **testicles**. See **Ovum**.

Spirochette: slender, spiral-shaped micro-organism that causes **syphilis**.

Sterility: abnormal condition of permanent **infertility**, resulting, for example, from birth defect, injury, dis-

ease, or surgical procedure. See
Fertility.

Symptom: a person's own sensation of some bodily process. Compare **Sign.**

Sympto-Thermic Method: a method of **natural family planning** that takes into account the **mucus** symptom, **basal body temperature,** and other signs of fertility.

Syphilis: a **venereal disease** transmitted by genital intercourse; caused by a **spirochette,** "Treponema pallidum." See page 46.

Testicles: male sex glands, in which **sperm** and **testosterone** are produced. See pages 24-25.

Testosterone: the male sex hormone responsible for secondary sex-characteristics of men. See page 10.

Trichomonas vaginitis: vaginal infection caused by a protozoan (one-celled animal), "Trichomonas vaginalis."

Tubal ligation: surgical procedure to bind or close the **fallopian tubes** so as to cause permanent **sterility** in a woman.

Urethra: tube through which urine flows from the bladder to the outside of the body.

Uterus (womb): pear-shaped female organ in which an infant grows during the period of **pregnancy.** See pages 20-22.

Vagina: the female organ of intercourse; also, the canal through which an infant passes at birth. See pages 21, 23-24.

Vaginitis: infection of the **vagina.**

Value: a belief that makes a difference in a person's behavior; a principle by which a decision is made.

Vas deferens: in men, the tube for transporting **sperm** from the **epididymis** to the **urethra.**

Vasectomy: a surgical excision of the **vas deferens** to produce permanent **sterility** in a man.

Venereal disease (VD): an infection spread by **genital relations** or contact.

Virginity: the state of not having freely engaged in genital activity or relations.

Virus: smallest, most primitive known form of life on earth.

Vulva: external parts of a woman's genital organs, enclosing the **clitoris,** the opening to the **vagina,** and the opening of the **urethra.** See pages 21, 25.

Wet dream: see **Nocturnal emission.**

Womb: see **Uterus.**

Yeast: see **Fungus.**

Zygote: the newly conceived baby from the moment of conception till **implantation** (about the first seven days of life). See **Blastocyst.**

Charles W. Norris, a graduate of Georgetown University School of Medicine, is a practicing obstetrician and gynecologist in Portland, Oregon. He has written and spoken on the subject of natural family planning in various forums. He is a member of the medical advisory committee of the World Organization Ovulation Method-Billings, U.S.A. He and his wife, Carol, have five children.

Jeanne Owen is a graduate of Portland State University, with a degree in anthropology and linguistics. She has been certified by W.O.O.M.B., U.S.A., to teach the Ovulation Method, and also by Natural Family Planning Teachers, Inc., of Oregon, to train instructors. She is a freelance writer. She and her husband, John, have two children.